INTERVENTIONAL CARDIOLOGY CLINICS

www.interventional.theclinics.com

Editor-in-Chief

MARVIN H. ENG

Chronic Total Occlusion

January 2021 • Volume 10 • Number 1

Editors

KATHLEEN E. KEARNEY
WILLIAM L. LOMBARDI

ELSEVIER

1600 John F. Kennedy Boulevard • Suite 1800 • Philadelphia, Pennsylvania, 19103-2899

http://www.theclinics.com

INTERVENTIONAL CARDIOLOGY CLINICS Volume 10, Number 1
January 2021 ISSN 2211-7458, ISBN-13: 978-0-323-79701-6

Editor: Joanna Collett
Developmental Editor: Donald Mumford

Interventional Cardiology Clinics (ISSN 2211-7458) is published quarterly by Elsevier Inc., 360 Park Avenue South, New York, NY 10010-1710. Months of issue are January, April, July, and October. Subscription prices are USD 209 per year for US individuals, USD 622 for US institutions, USD 100 per year for US students, USD 209 per year for Canadian individuals, USD 638 for Canadian institutions, USD 100 per year for Canadian students, USD 296 per year for international individuals, USD 638 for international institutions, and USD 150 per year for international students. To receive student/resident rate, orders must be accompanied by name of affiliated institution, date of term, and the *signature* of program/residency coordinator on institution letterhead. Orders will be billed at individual rate until proof of status is received. Foreign air speed delivery is included in all *Clinics* subscription prices. All prices are subject to change without notice. **POSTMASTER:** Send address changes to *Interventional Cardiology Clinics*, Elsevier Health Sciences Division, Subscription Customer Service, 3251 Riverport Lane, Maryland Heights, MO 63043. **Customer Service: Telephone: 1-800-654-2452** (U.S. and Canada); **1-314-447-8871** (outside U.S. and Canada). **Fax: 1-314-447-8029. E-mail: journalscustomerservice-usa@elsevier.com (for print support); journalsonlinesupport-usa@elsevier.com (for online support)**.

Reprints. For copies of 100 or more of articles in this publication, please contact the Commercial Reprints Department, Elsevier Inc., 360 Park Avenue South, New York, NY 10010-1710. Tel.: 212-633-3874; Fax: 212-633-3820; E-mail: reprints@elsevier.com.

Printed in the United States of America.

CONTRIBUTORS

EDITOR-IN-CHIEF

MARVIN H. ENG, MD
Director of Research for the Center of Structural Heart Disease, Structural Heart Disease Fellowship Director, Henry Ford Hospital, Detroit, Michigan, USA

EDITORS

KATHLEEN E. KEARNEY, MD
Assistant Professor, Division of Cardiology, University of Washington, Seattle, Washington, USA

WILLIAM L. LOMBARDI, MD
Professor, Division of Cardiology, University of Washington, Seattle, Washington, USA

AUTHORS

YOUSIF AHMAD, MD, PhD
Division of Cardiology, Center for Interventional Vascular Therapy, New York Presbyterian Hospital/Columbia University Irving Medical Center, New York, New York, USA

ZIAD A. ALI, MD, DPhil
Division of Cardiology, Center for Interventional Vascular Therapy, New York Presbyterian Hospital/Columbia University Irving Medical Center, Clinical Trials Center, Cardiovascular Research Foundation, New York, New York, USA; St. Francis Hospital, Roslyn, New York, USA

KATRINA A.E.L. BIDWELL, MD
Cardiology Fellow, Medical University of South Carolina, Charleston, South Carolina, USA

AMY CHENEY, MD
Interventional Cardiology Fellow, Department of Cardiology, University of Washington Medical Center, Seattle, Washington, USA

STEWART BENTON, Jr, MD
Interventional Cardiology, Director of CTO and Complex Coronary Disease, Wellspan York Hospital, York, Pennsylvania, USA

RHIAN E. DAVIES, DO, MS
Acting Instructor/Advanced Interventional Cardiology Fellow, Department of Cardiology, University of Washington Medical Center, Seattle, Washington, USA

KATHRYN DAWSON, MD
Interventional Cardiology Fellow, Department of Cardiology, University of Washington Medical Center, Seattle, Washington, USA

KHADY N. FALL, MD
Division of Cardiology, Center for Interventional Vascular Therapy, New York Presbyterian Hospital/Columbia University Irving Medical Center, New York, New York, USA

J. AARON GRANTHAM, MD
Associate Professor of Medicine, Saint Luke's Mid America Heart Institute, University of Missouri-Kansas City, Kansas City, Missouri, USA

ALLISON B. HALL, MD
Interventional Cardiologist, Clinical Assistant Professor of Medicine, Eastern Health/Memorial University of Newfoundland, C/O Cardiology Consultants, St. John's, Newfoundland, Canada

RAVI S. HIRA, MD
Associate Professor of Medicine, Department of Cardiology, University of Washington Medical Center, Seattle, Washington, USA

TAISHI HIRAI, MD
Assistant Professor of Clinical Medicine, University of Missouri, Columbia, Missouri, USA

ALLEN JEREMIAS, MD
Clinical Trials Center, Cardiovascular Research Foundation, New York, New York, USA; St. Francis Hospital, Roslyn, New York, USA

DIMITRI KARMPALIOTIS, MD, PhD
Division of Cardiology, Center for Interventional Vascular Therapy, New York Presbyterian Hospital/Columbia University Irving Medical Center, New York, New York, USA

AJAY J. KIRTANE, MD
Division of Cardiology, Center for Interventional Vascular Therapy, New York Presbyterian Hospital/Columbia University Irving Medical Center, New York, New York, USA

AKIKO MAEHARA, MD
Division of Cardiology, Center for Interventional Vascular Therapy, New York Presbyterian Hospital/Columbia University Irving Medical Center, Clinical Trials Center, Cardiovascular Research Foundation, New York, New York, USA

ANBUKARASI MARAN, MD
Associate Professor of Medicine, Medical University of South Carolina, Charleston, South Carolina, USA

STEVEN P. MARSO, MD
Executive Medical Director, Cardiovascular Service Line, HCA Midwest Health, Kansas City, Missouri, USA

JAMES M. McCABE, MD
Associate Professor of Medicine, Department of Cardiology, University of Washington Medical Center, Seattle, Washington, USA

MARGARET B. McENTEGART, MD, PhD
Department of Cardiology, Golden Jubilee National Hospital, Glasgow, United Kingdom

MICHAEL MEGALY, MD, MS
Clinical Instructor of Medicine, University of Arizona College of Medicine Phoenix, Phoenix, Arizona, USA

GARY S. MINTZ, MD
Division of Cardiology, Center for Interventional Vascular Therapy, New York Presbyterian Hospital/Columbia University Irving Medical Center, New York, New York, USA

JEFFREY W. MOSES, MD
Division of Cardiology, Center for Interventional Vascular Therapy, New York Presbyterian Hospital/Columbia University Irving Medical Center, New York, New York, USA; St. Francis Hospital, Roslyn, New York, USA

WILLIAM J. NICHOLSON, MD
Interventional Cardiology, Director, Complex Coronary and Cardiac Intervention, Emory University, Atlanta, Georgia, USA

ANJA ØKSNES, MD
Department of Cardiology, Haukeland University Hospital, Bergen, Norway

ASHISH PERSHAD, MD, MS
Associate Professor of Medicine, University of Arizona College of Medicine Phoenix, Phoenix, Arizona, USA

MEGHA PRASAD, MD, MS
Division of Cardiology, Center for Interventional Vascular Therapy, New York Presbyterian Hospital/Columbia University Irving Medical Center, New York, New York, USA

JEREMY D. RIER, DO
Acting Instructor/Advanced Interventional Cardiology Fellow, Department of Cardiology, University of Washington Medical Center, Seattle, Washington, USA

STÉPHANE RINFRET, MD, SM, FRCP(C), FSCAI, FACC
Division of Cardiology, Department of Medicine, Director, Interventional Cardiology, Associate Professor of Medicine, McGill

University, McGill University Health Centre, Montreal, Quebec, Canada

EVAN SHLOFMITZ, DO
Clinical Trials Center, Cardiovascular Research Foundation, New York, New York, USA; St. Francis Hospital, Roslyn, New York, USA

CRAIG A. THOMPSON, MD, MMSc
Director, Interventional Cardiology, NYU Langone Health System, Lead, Cardiac Catheterization Laboratories, NYU Langone Health System, Director, Cardiac Catheterization Laboratories, NYU Langone-Tisch Hospital, Professor of Medicine, New York University School of Medicine, New York, New York, USA

JENNIFER A. TREMMEL, MD, MS
Associate Professor of Medicine (Cardiovascular), Stanford University Medical Center, Stanford, California, USA

LUIZ F. YBARRA, MD, PhD, MBA
Director, CTO PCI Program, Assistant Professor of Medicine, London Health Sciences Centre, Schulich School of Medicine & Dentistry, Western University, London, Ontario, Canada

R. MICHAEL WYMAN, MD, FACC
Director, Cardiovascular Interventional Research, Torrance Memorial Medical Center, Torrance, California, USA

CONTENTS

Chronic total occlusions remain among the most technically challenging lesions
to treat percutaneously. Limitations of 2-dimensional angiography may further
hinder successful treatment of these lesions. Intravascular ultrasound has a key
role in percutaneous recanalization for a chronic total occlusion by providing
key lesion characteristics, facilitating guidewire crossing, elucidating the intraplaque or extralaque path of the guidewire, optimizing lesion preparation,
guiding stenting and identifying suboptimal results. Live visualization of the
guidewire during crossing may reduce extraplaque wire tracking. This review
describes the practical uses of intravascular imaging for commonly encountered scenarios when treating chronic total occlusions.

Selected patients with coronary chronic total occlusion (CTO) benefit with respect
to symptoms, quality of life, ischemia reduction, and potentially longevity among
other benefits. CTO lesions tend to be the most technically challenging for practicing interventional cardiologists to deliver a successful and safe result and clinical
experience for a given patient. The Hybrid algorithm for CTO percutaneous coronary intervention and the subsequent subalgorithms for focused technical challenges have a standardized process and provide a consistent platform for
optimized patient care, medical education, and clinical investigation in patients
challenged with total occlusion and complex coronary disease.

Coronary perforation is a relatively common and potentially lethal complication
of percutaneous coronary intervention for chronic total occlusion. Approximately one-half of these perforations require treatment, and there are certain
features that can signify a more high-risk perforation. Perforation management
depends on the perforation site, the severity of the perforation, and the hemodynamic status of the patients. Large vessel perforations are generally treated
with a covered stent, while small vessel perforations are generally treated with
embolization. Because there are certain mechanisms known to increase the risk
of perforation, steps to minimize these occurrences in the fist place are best.

▶ Video content accompanies this article at http://www.interventional.theclinics.com.

Coronary perforations during chronic total occlusion percutaneous coronary
intervention (CTO PCI) is a most frequent major complication and the incidence is significantly higher compared with non-CTO PCI. Patients with prior
history of coronary bypass have more major adverse events when perforation
occurs compared with patients without prior bypass surgery. In this article,
the authors discuss the unique challenges in identification and timely treatment
of perforations in patients with prior bypass surgery.

Dual access for chronic total occlusion percutaneous coronary intervention is considered best practice by many experts. There are 2 access sites: radial and femoral. Both accesses have important advantages and disadvantages. Determining the ratio risk/benefit–efficacy/safety of each access for each patient in a specific procedure should be based on procedural and clinical variables. Given the safety benefit and the minimal procedural disadvantages, radial access should be the standard approach, especially in procedures of low complexity and in patients at high risk of vascular complications. Nonetheless, mastering both approaches is important because they are needed in multiple occasions.

Coronary artery disease continues to advance resulting in the development of high-risk percutaneous interventions. This includes treatment of patients with multivessel disease, unprotected left main, acute myocardial infarction complicated by cardiogenic shock, and depressed left ventricular ejection fraction. As a result, mechanical circulatory support devices have evolved but require an understanding of patient hemodynamics, device mechanics, and access management. Trial data regarding device selection are limited by inclusion of cardiogenic shock patients, and observational studies are conflicted by selection bias, site familiarity with devices, and complication management; therefore, clinical judgment is required to treat high-risk patients appropriately.

Complex coronary artery intervention stresses the limits of both the operator's skills as well as the equipment being used for the procedure. This article is focused on avoiding, recognizing and dealing with device failure and gear entrapment during complex coronary intervention. The operator must understand how to avoid these complications by understanding the limits of devices and the need for adequate vessel preparation. This article focuses on giving the reader an algorithmic approach to recognizing when device failure/entrapment occurs and what specific maneuvers can be done to retrieve different devices and equipment safely.

CHRONIC TOTAL OCCLUSION

FORTHCOMING ISSUES

April 2021
Mechanical Circulatory Support
Brian O'Neill, *Editor*

July 2021
State of the Art in STEMI Care
Ravi S. Hira, *Editor*

RECENT ISSUES

October 2020
Key Trials of the Decade
Matthew J. Price, *Editor*

July 2020
Renal Disease and Coronary, Peripheral and
Structural Interventions
Hitinder S. Gurm, *Editor*

THE CLINICS ARE NOW AVAILABLE ONLINE!

RELATED SERIES

Cardiology Clinics
Cardiac Electrophysiology Clinics
Heart Failure Clinics

Access your subscription at:
www.theclinics.com

FOREWORD

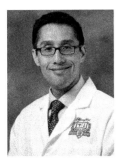

Marvin H. Eng, MD
Consulting Editor

We are pleased to introduce this issue of *Interventional Cardiology Clinics* discussing the art of chronic total occlusion (CTO) percutaneous coronary intervention (PCI). Evolution of CTO PCI has been one of the most exciting and provocative developments in medicine in the past decade. Consistent with the accelerating advances in interventional cardiology, operator skill and medical product development have converged to make CTO PCI a niche specialty.

While CTOs have been a common problem through the history of PCI, only recently have the tools and skills been refined enough to tackle this difficult challenge. First, a thorough understanding of the lesion, coronary collaterals, and plaque consistency is required to plan the procedure. In addition, extensive knowledge and comfort with working inside the subintimal space are needed since subintimal dissection is commonplace. Difficulty with microcatheter and stent delivery is frequent and may require tools such as atherectomy and other special devices reserved for experts. Suboptimal surgical candidates are often referred for CTO PCI as an alternative. Their comorbidities, length, and complexity of the procedures may require the use of mechanical circulatory support to facilitate the procedure. Finally, adventitial breach is not uncommon, making perforation management fundamentally essential for survival. This quantum leap in interventional cardiology requires significant dedication to training and practice.

This issue of *Interventional Cardiology Clinics* has been edited by 2 luminaries in the field of CTO PCI. We congratulate Drs. Lombardi and Kearney for updating us on the most cutting-edge advances in PCI. Readership should find this issue to be an enlightening and practical guide for sharpening their PCI knowledge.

Marvin H. Eng, MD
Center of Structural Heart Disease
Henry Ford Hospital
Clara Ford Pavilion RM 434
2799 West Grand Boulevard
Detroit, MI 48202, USA

E-mail address:
meng1@hfhs.org

Intervent Cardiol Clin 10 (2021) xiii
https://doi.org/10.1016/j.iccl.2020.10.002
2211-7458/21/© 2020 Published by Elsevier Inc.

INTRODUCTION

The Self Work of Becoming a CTO Operator

Thy word is a lamp onto my feet and a light unto my path

—Psalm 119:10

In this article, I only have my experiences to share. I have not researched much for this article, and I cite no literature. This will be a most unusual article. At times, the content is too vulnerable for my comfort level and will also probably make you, the reader, a bit uncomfortable as well. And maybe that's ok. But it is my story. It is my truth.

TAKE A STEP. ONE STEP ONLY

The path you have chosen is hard but yet known. It is narrow and well-traveled, not by everyone but by many. Of these many, there are some who know this single track very well. They travel often and far. If you seek their advice, they are willing and able to help.

This journey begins with a single step and ends only when you croak, or quit. (Don't let others unduly influence you to do the latter.) Once you have chosen to take the first step, your only job is to decide when to take the next. This journey has a beginning but no defined ending. There is no turnaround point, and the journey does not circle back to the beginning. On this pathway, you will both succeed and fail, sometimes in epic fashion. You will feel competent and incompetent. You will help and hurt. You will have a constellation of emotions linked to your work. You will do self-work that will help you not only in your cath lab life but also in your personal life. You will meet others who will encourage you and those who will discourage you. Learn from both. Don't be too swayed by either.

Along the way, I encourage you to work hard, to be curious, to have a zest for knowledge, to be open to new ways of doing things, to not get stuck in your old ways of thinking and working in the cath lab, to be vigilant while working on patients, to remain committed, to learn both cognitive and technical skills, and to frequently reassess your interest and capabilities. I know this is a lot, but it is all really important. *Also, enjoy your journey.*

This issue is a testament to the concept that the trade craft of CTO PCI can be learned. It can be taught, and it can be replicated. You will feel lonely during very deep emotional valleys along the way. But you don't have to be alone. Others are available to you. Phone a friend is alive and well among the CTO community. Others have similar experiences and can navigate you out of these valleys.

There is self-work to be done. This may seem strange, to think of self-work to do just to learn a new medical procedure, but I would encourage you to keep an open mind about this along the way. Becoming a capable CTO operator may be one of the hardest things you tackle in your professional life. The journey at times is steep and unforgiving, and it is long; remember there is a beginning but no end.

It is good for all of us in the CTO space to remember no one owns this pathway. It rests on public ground. There are folks who have discovered the route and described its known course. They have done very fine work. And, I believe the path remains both incompletely explored and incompletely described. There is meaningful work to do.

SELF-IDENTIFY (BUT NOT SOLELY) AS A CTO OPERATOR

After you have taken your first step, please publicly declare your intentions to become a capable CTO operator. This avoids the ambiguity of whether you are on the path or not. This is a binary decision. Are you in or are you out? It can be confusing to self and others until you publicly commit to this journey. This is a seemingly small ask but has profound implications. You need to double down and internally commit because it will drive your behavior and the behavior of people around you. With your declaration, others will invest in your development. Make yourself available.

I wasn't deliberate about this step early on, and I believe this singular nonaction resulted in a delay of my CTO development. I did not self-identify as

Intervent Cardiol Clin 10 (2021) xv–xxiii
https://doi.org/10.1016/j.iccl.2020.09.010

a CTO operator for quite some time after starting my journey. To declare was risky for me. I had accomplished much in my professional career and what if this was a failure. Would I then be a failure? I will discuss this more later in this article, but I lost my center and I was drawn far into the extreme thinking that if I failed as a CTO operator, then I was a failure. Therefore, I hedged my bet for a while. I would encourage to not take this detour on the CTO journey. It is a long way back to the pathway. This detour is a dead end. Declare you are on the path.

Others recognized that I didn't identify as a CTO operator, and this was brought to my attention several years ago. After a CTO course, a few CTO operators and I gathered around a table for dinner. (Note how I wrote this: "CTO operators and I." This was how I thought at the time. There were CTO operators, and there was me. There was not an us. There was not a we. There was a them and me.) I didn't belong, even though at the time I was definitely on the CTO pathway, probably for 2 to 3 years. At the table were several master operators, me, and 2 to 3 attendees of the course. Soon after sitting, the conversation zeroed in on the latest concepts related to CTO PCI. During the course of discussion, it became clear, at least to 1 individual, that I didn't perceive myself as part of the larger-collective CTO community. Unknowingly, I was asking questions but using the pronouns of you and you guys rather than a collective we. It may seem small, but internally I didn't feel as though I had crossed some imaginary milestone on my journey to be "voted" in or worthy of using the collective we when in the presence of CTO operators. In my midsentence, I was interrupted and confronted with something I wasn't even aware of. "Marso, why are you using 'you guys' and 'you'? You are part of the community." He went on to say, "you have chosen to walk the path. You are in. Cash the check and quit feeling like an outsider." I am paraphrasing the words, but contextually this was the message from an astute listener and colleague. It was then and remains now good advice.

At the time I didn't realize the implications of not feeling part of the larger collective. But now I have come to believe that you will deprive yourself of support if you take this detour. You will also be delayed in acquiring essential new information and new technical skills. If you act like me, you will want to set some arbitrary milestone like doing 40 retrogrades or your first high-end blind stick and swap (or whatever) before declaring or self-identifying. Please resist this temptation and let it be known to yourself and others that you have chosen this path and that you feel worthy of identifying with us and to make yourself available. This simple act will facilitate your development in ways that are unpredictable to you.

Declaring can be vulnerable for some of you. I get it. Once you put it out there, then what? What if I fail? What if I am not as good in the lab as I need to be? What if I am not even better at CTOs than a non-CTO operator? This list of "not good enoughs" goes on and on. What if I decide this really isn't for me and I decide to get off this journey? Then what? I get all this self-talk. But if you declare and engage, there are ways through all of this. Others have navigated the path.

A word of caution. There is a balance here. There will be a temptation for you to overidentify as a CTO operator. You will be very committed to this journey, and you may tend to make this too big of a thing in your life. *It is healthy to identify with CTO operators but not solely as a CTO operator.* This latter extreme is dangerous. That is to identify solely as a CTO operator. Your self-worth, your importance, and your essence are not defined by how good you are in the cath lab. It is not defined by opening chronic total occlusions. Do not be deceived otherwise. You will experience great successes on this journey, and you will suffer through epic failures. If you stay on this journey long enough, both will happen. Do not be defined by either of these 2 extremes. It is super important that you understand this concept early and guard against this temptation often. I have seen this play out among friends and colleagues (and lived through it myself) many times in my life.

Not long ago I shared a ride to the airport with 2 individuals; both had been on the CTO pathway for many years. A colleague shared that he was under enormous pressure to succeed as he had just started a new position at a high-profile institution to lead their CTO program. There was just no room for failure here. All eyes are on me. There is just no space for not being good enough at this place. There is no room for anything but success after success after success. Are we still quoting CTO success rates at 90%? I need to be better than that. That is the national average. This place isn't average. I am not average. I am at a leading institution, and they picked me. I need to be better than that. The weight of the world squarely rested on his shoulders. We all felt it. Hell, the taxicab driver felt it through the Plexiglas. I believe he thought that the outcome of his early days here would define him as a person for a long time to come. If he failed here, then he was a failure. If he succeeded, then he was successful. He was under so much pressure, and it was affecting every facet of his life. It was affecting his health, his free time, his family, his joy. Stress oozed into every part of his life, and on that day, was oozing out of him. He was oozy. He was overpressurized.

DEPRESSURIZE (FOR COMFORT SAKE)

Billie Jean King is often quoted as saying (feeling) pressure is a privilege. While this may be true, we all know how much pressure we dial up (in the inflation device as in life) is optional. Too much pressure will lead to a cascade of events that can end in catastrophe (perforation of the proximal LAD and implosion at the midpoint of life). Too little pressure, and nothing gets done. Pressure is titratable and needs to be optimized.

I enjoy cycling the gravel roads of Kansas these days. I am certainly not well versed in all the technicalities of cycling. However, I am learning. Years ago, it was a commonly held belief that to optimize speed and efficiency, cyclists needed highly pressurized (100 atm) and very narrow tires (19 mm). The dogma at the time was that very narrow, highly pressurized tires were integral to being fast and efficient. It turns out this just isn't true. Within an acceptable range, there is no association between tire width and tire pressure with performance as measured by speed and efficiency. What is clear to everyone who rides is that wider tires at lower pressure is a lot more comfortable to ride especially when riding on long rough terrain, like the gravel farm roads of Kansas. So, 19-mm tires inflated to 100 atm have been replaced with 40-mm tires at 40 atm with very little loss of efficiency. I think we have covered that the CTO pathway, like Kansas gravel roads, is long and rocky. So, I would suggest that you depressurize and widen your tires. Your outcomes will not suffer, and you will be much more comfortable (and less oozy) along the way. Recognizing that you are overpressurized is the first step. Finding healthy ways to depressurize is your next.

STAY CENTERED

At the time we were in the cab to the airport with our oozy friend, I hadn't done enough self-work to be of much help to him or anyone else for that matter. I think I said something to the effect of "yeah, that sucks" and then changed the subject. So helpful. However, I could certainly relate to what he was saying. I had felt it many times before in my life. I had gotten sucked into the paradigm of doing something successful and then equating that to me as a person being a success. Similarly, if I failed at something important, then I was a failure. We are all susceptible to equating an outcome of one of our activities to our self-worth. Be careful with this. Guard against this. If left unchecked, this can lead to a cataclysmic ending to your journey.

I have fallen prey to this type of thinking so many times in my life, and if left unchecked, I am 1 step away from doing this again. That is, to overvalue a priority activity. This is a slippery slope and can sneak up on you. Be careful.

Perhaps the best advice I have read that helps to avoid this pitfall was written by Bob Buford. In his book *Halftime: Moving from Success to Significance*, he does a nice job of summarizing how one can balance (both great successes and epic failures) the extremes of life in a healthy way. Chapter 11, "Finding the Center and Staying There," notes, "… it is important to be deliberate about finding and holding in comfortable balance the creative tension that is the reality of life." It is important to identify the extremes of your life where we are often caught and then resolve internally how we will deal with this great tension in a way that is not self-destructive. The great tensions of your life may differ from others, but there are surely similarities for us all: family versus work, charity versus wealth, success versus failure, keeping personal perspective in the face of great success and monumental failures. Buford suggests that we should not perceive these tensions in our life negatively but rather find ways to reduce the stress of life by learning how to hold this paradox in our mind and life at the same time. Find peace in the fact that, while we live on this earth, we will never solve these tensions. They will always be there, and this tension is ok. Balance the extremes by remaining centered in your life and in your choices and in your belief systems. Stay there and don't rebel against or move rapidly toward the extremes. Recognize that your life will toggle quickly between anxiety and boredom, success and failure, and many other extremes. Recognize that for what it is. Don't get sucked into either. Hold both. Don't be defined by either. That is not to say there aren't important lessons to be learned from the extremes of life. There most certainly are. But these extremes do not define you.

Being sucked into the extremes of your life is destabilizing. Stay centered and in the moment. People can hold extreme tension surrounding them in life and be perfectly calm and peaceful and present and centered. You can hold both realities and yet still remain true to your core beliefs. This is important self-work to start and continue to do until you die. Don't quit this work even if you choose to step off of the CTO pathway. This transcends CTOs.

There will be many extremes on your journey. Below I mention two:

BENCHMARKING YOUR PERFORMANCE TO OTHERS

Observing others' skill sets and striving to be better can be highly motivating but if left unchecked can lead to thoughts of never being good enough. As you watch and learn from others, I would encourage you to dial up your specificity thinking and dial down your generalizability thinking. Picture you are at a live CTO case conference and there is a top CTO operator working on a large screen. She is good. Better than you. No doubt about it. Generalized thinking would be that person is really good, much better than me. I am not good enough. Time to quit! I am out. Switch from this to very specific thinking. She does a great job of executing a high-end stick and swap when there is an occlusive subintimal hematoma at a bifurcation. I need to go find her after the course, and figure out what she is doing different because I need to work on that aspect of my journey. Go specific and compartmentalize your talents and your deficiencies. Don't go general here. It works.

SUCCESS AND FAILURE

Feel the joy and elation with an epic success. Celebrate the wins and know this is but 1 facet or 1 extreme of being a CTO operator. Emotions are not good or bad, they just are, and they can teach you a lesson (or two). A well-centered person will also recognize that failure and turmoil are just around the corner. Hold both. Don't overvalue (or undervalue) either. This is not to say that successes shouldn't be celebrated. They should. And this isn't to say there aren't priceless life lessons with failure. There are. Just be careful to not let that single moment in time overdefine you as a person or operator. Stay centered.

PACE AND TOLERANCE

Your journey is neither a sprint nor an endurance race. It is not a race at all.

When I reread the Psalmist's verse, "Thy word is a lamp onto my feet and a light unto my path," I picture a small candlelight that illuminates the next step of the journey. It need not (and most certainly does not) highlight the entire path, only the next step. I envision the light also identifying the danger spots and the wrong turns. I would encourage you to use the resources available to you (the light) to illuminate your next step. It is not helpful to get too far down the road in your thinking or obsessing about the ground already covered.

It is also natural to want to quicken your pace along the way. Be careful with this. Make sure you have mastered your current step and ensure you are on stable ground before you identify and take your next step. Try to resist quickening the pace for any reason. From time to time, you may feel a strong desire to move faster than is natural or safe along the pathway. You may feel a desire to move more quickly to get better faster. You may feel compelled to catch up to a group in front of you. You may have patients who present to you with very complex problems and you are not quite there on the pathway yet. You may feel the need to grow your CTO practice faster. It is natural to want to get better. And you are wired to get better just as fast as you can. It is difficult (and at times unsafe) to artificially quicken your pace. Your mind and thinking will get ahead of your cognitive and technical development. Try to be aware of this tension as you make your journey down the CTO pathway. Be patient with yourself.

There is a relationship between how fast we move on this journey and the risk of moving faster. I've come to think differently about this because of what a friend of mine who is a Chief Financial Officer for a large corporation has taught me. He has taught me much about the concept of pace and tolerance. Through his financial lens, he talks about the rate of business growth as a function of an individual's (or corporation's) tolerance for risk. He articulates pace or rate of business growth is proportionate to risk tolerance or downside risk of losing money. As I thought about this proportional relationship, I have come to believe that this applies to many things in life, including our CTO journey.

The pace of your CTO journey is at least in part proportional to risk tolerance. As you think about this relationship, I want you to think about your personal risk tolerance, the risk tolerance of patients you serve, the risk tolerance of colleagues, and the risk tolerance of your institution. Your safe pace is governed by the risk tolerance of these people and institutions. You should consider each as you progress down your CTO pathway.

Pace is proportional (at least in part) to risk tolerance
Your Risk Tolerance
Your tolerance for risk is a major consideration. You have chosen to learn a new skill that will place you in very difficult situations. You have chosen to help people who have chronic stable but often progressive symptoms. Yet, CTOs are universally elective procedures. You have assessed that the

patient's symptoms warrant a higher-risk procedure to minimize symptoms and improve their quality of life. Your goal is to help, but at times you will harm. Many people are not wired to take on this clinical challenge. Their default is to do nothing (often an error of omission). This is an intensely personal decision to begin this pathway, to start this clinical practice. If you have made it to this article, you clearly are wired to help these types of individuals.

The next level of self-work is less obvious and thus a bit harder to discern. You are wired to help, but there are other variables, other risks to you and your journey that need consideration. What is your risk tolerance to fail? How many times will you allow yourself to fail and still get back up and keep going? When performing CTO PCIs, you will fail safe, and you will fail and cause harm. These will feel very different to you. These 2 failure modes will affect your thinking and emotions very differently. I would encourage you to understand how you will react to both of these failure modes. How often these happen to you may define whether you're willing to continue on this journey. You'll need to pick yourself up, dust off, process the lessons learned from failing, and move on with your journey. Over time, you will accommodate to both failing and succeeding (by being depressurized and staying centered). Along the way, you will develop strategies to fail safe and you will recognize maneuvers you are about to make that could result in both failure and harm. You will learn. But it does take time. The pace of your journey is a function of your risk tolerance.

As I write this section, there is so much more to share about your risk tolerance. This content would probably result in a separate article. Briefly, there are additional risks to you lurking on your pathway. You will have thoughts that you are inadequate. You will watch other operators work, and many will be more capable and more proficient than you are at that point in time. You will fail when you thought you should have succeeded. Others will comment directly or indirectly on your performance. In the beginning, these comments will be predominantly negative and discouraging. When these events occur (and they will), you may have feelings that you are inadequate. You may feel that you are not good enough. Your thinking may lead you to the conclusion that you should stop this journey. We have all experienced this. This is predictable. I would be surprised if this doesn't happen to you along the way. This is all a natural part of progression. Anticipate these things. When you feel this way, phone a CTO friend. We have all reached out. Most of us answer our phones when we are free, day or night. We have definitely all been there. We will all be there again.

Patient Risk

There are other strategies available to manage patient risk. But I wanted to share 1 practice that I think is helpful, at least to me. I would encourage you to personally see, evaluate, and perform informed consent on CTO patients. This allows me the opportunity to individualize the likelihood of success, the likelihood of failure, and the likelihood of complications given the patient's anatomy, frailty, and comorbidities. Moreover, it allows me to develop a one-on-one relationship with not only the patient but also the family. This may seem obvious but as you develop a CTO practice, a program, and maybe as a proctor (to colleagues in your practice and other CTO operators), this will be harder to do over time. To this day, I try to avoid walking into the cath lab without meeting the patient and the family and providing a discussion of what we will be doing. This practice helps me manage my perceptions of risk.

Colleagues' Risk Tolerance

It is uncomfortable and true that others are watching you. People notice, especially early on in your journey. They will form opinions, and more often than not, will comment, not directly to you, but about you to others. This triangulation is problematic. Depending on the prework you have done to set up others' expectations of your development, this chatter can derail your development and the development of your CTO practice/program. Why I think this happens is a very long discussion, but this does happen. The likelihood for you to navigate this is dependent on your knowledge of their risk tolerance and their acceptance that you are the right person to develop the CTO program. In addition, it is important that colleagues believe that a CTO program is needed and that your approach to personal development and transparency is genuine. Below are a couple of my suggestions to help navigate other people's perceptions of risk tolerance.

- Do your prework. Develop the cognitive and technical skills appropriate to the cases you are doing.
- Make it public that you are a CTO operator and doing the work.
- Be consistent and honest in your assessment of symptoms and indications.
- If possible, invite referring doctors to the lab and/or invite them to co-scrub.

Be transparent with both your early successes and your early failures. One of the mistakes I witness is operators who celebrate and share early successes but deep-six the failures. Be transparent with both. Learn from both.

- Be kind and humble as you progress. You will likely develop well beyond the capabilities of your colleagues.
- Be available to colleagues when they need help in the cath lab with non-CTO problems. You can establish a deep sense of loyalty when you help another non-CTO operator fix a problem they have caused or a problem they encounter but cannot fix.

Institutional Risk Tolerance

Many cardiovascular institutions have a very ingrained culture about high-risk, high-reward procedures. Of course, every institution would love to be profiled on the nightly news to discuss how their team of 8 surgeons performed a very heroic high-risk procedure that saved the life of a young child. But that is not what we are talking about with CTO PCI. It's entirely different for an institution to take on a very common cardiology procedure that has a steep and long learning curve, is associated with higher (than acceptable) risk to patients, and occurs frequently (10%–20% of all PCI). In the era of public reporting, this is problematic for many hospital administrators and physician leaders. If your institution is risk averse and has not fully bought into the risk-reward paradigm of CTO PCI, this may be an insurmountable problem. In fact, this can be, based upon my personal experience, a perfect storm if you are early in your development and are still calibrating your pace-tolerance curve. It can also grow to be a problem if you are a very senior CTO operator who is referred in the hardest cases from around the region or country. This institutional misalignment sometimes cannot be fixed.

I lived through this very difficult experience. I know others with similar stories. Early in my CTO development, I was at a very risk-averse institution where it became clear that the neither the hospital leadership nor the academic administrators had a tolerance for cardiovascular complications following CTO PCI. A retroperitoneal bleed and a coronary perforation that required surgical repair and bypass were deal breakers. I did not understand, as well as I do now, the importance of the pace-tolerance curve. I overshot the risk tolerance for the institution (and likely colleagues). I may have never been able to dial down risk to an acceptable level for this institution, to be honest. It became mutually understood that I would need to move institutions if I was going to continue to develop as a CTO PCI operator. This, by the way, turned out to be one of the best things for my development. However, it was a painful experience at the time. I now practice at an institution where we have a developed a CTO program that is sustainable and growing in volume and case complexity. At the time, the move was personally painful but necessary. This was an incredibly difficult, humbling, and painful time in my professional life. Looking back, I learned an enormous amount about the CTO journey. A former mentor of mine taught me that you need to have the courage of your convictions. Acting on your convictions can be painful in the short term but rewarding in the long term.

Risk tolerance is not the only driver of pace. Your commitment and dedication to acquiring new information and new technical skills are key ingredients to your success is a CTO operator. The work ethic of accomplished CTO operators is palpable. Your work ethic is critically important for your journey. I do not want to dwell on this fact, but I would be remiss to not clearly state that your effort and willingness to work both in the cath lab and in preparing for the cath lab are foundational. Lifelong learning for CTO PCI has little to do with maintenance of certification or continuing medical education points. Lifelong learning is however the CTO PCI journey.

FLUENCY MILESTONES

You will become a competent CTO operator over time. You will cross major milestones without you even knowing they existed. I want to share a couple of these with you.

Your competency will of course be evident in your daily practice and the cases you are taking on. Your volume and case complexity will increase month over month and year over year. Your cases will morph into a practice, and your practice into a program. When you evolve, so will your team and colleagues. When you wrap up your career, you will likely leave behind a very robust and sustainable program.

You will cross milestones on your CTO journey, and many of these milestones will go unrecognized by you. Others who are fluent in this subspecialty will probably notice. True experts in a field have the ability to discern the good from great and the great from the elite. The ability to discern performance among highly trained individuals is acquired over time. Your progress will be noticed by them for sure.

CTO Dialect

The language used among CTO operators is different. There is a CTO dialect. When I was first learning, I found it difficult to follow along while watching a live CTO case, but it was way harder to follow 2 proficient CTO operators talk about a case. There were just too many new words and concepts. Their speech was fast. The words were new. The visual images came too slowly in my mind. As one image slowly resolved to clarity (a blind stick and swap), they had flipped to GuideLiner-assisted reverse cart through an epicardial collateral. The concepts were just too new, and the cases were just too complex to follow. They tossed the hybrid algorithm around like a garden salad. It was crazy hard to follow. They understood each other. That was obvious. I was lost.

Not very long ago, I called up a friend and we were talking about a case, and he interrupted and said, "Marso, you talk CTO now." (Check. Another milestone crossed. I didn't even know there was a CTO dialect milestone. But alas there is.) True experts discern.

Becoming facile with CTO procedures will bring forth a CTO dialect in you. The change will occur slowly and may well go unnoticed by you. By the way, when you become fluent in the CTO dialect and need to communicate with non-CTO operators, they have no idea what you are talking about. Which is ok if you don't care that they are not following. If you want to be understood, you will need to slow down and define every step. You will likely also need to draw a lot of pictures.

Cath Lab Performance

Competent CTO operators can rapidly identify CTO operators by standing next to them in the cath lab doing a case. A CTO operator can identify other facile operators in less than 5 to 10 minutes of starting a case. The setup is different. The thinking is different. The gear is different. The amount of time spent trying a strategy to complete a task in the lab is less. It is a different case approach. There is no hiding from that. There is no faking your work in the lab when faced with a CTO. It is a humbling procedure. As you develop your skills, your colleagues will not be able to keep up with either your thinking or the pace of your technical work. Please invest in your assistants. They are vital to your success and the safety of your patients. They can support you if you invest enough time and energy into their development.

CTO Dreaming

I am going to receive an enormous amount of grief for this section. My only hope is that nobody reads this article, and if they start, they will lose interest long before getting to this section.

Dreaming in a foreign language is considered a sign of fluency. You've probably heard people talk about the moment when they started to dream in a foreign language. It's often considered a sign of fluency.

Dreaming in a second language is a sign of fluency. I have no idea how many CTO operators dream about CTO procedures. I have been too embarrassed to ask. But I started CTO dreaming some time ago. My CTO dreams are a bit weird though. CTO dreaming is probably a sign of CTO fluency or at least a sincere preoccupation with CTOs.

Treetop CTO Dreaming

In a recurring dream, I stand on a small platform (probably the base of operations) a hundred feet above a steep rocky hillside (risky). The platform is wedged between 2 small tree limbs (not a lot of space to maneuver) in the ceiling of a dense forest canopy several hundred feet above the closest piece of solid ground. The platform sways yet seems sturdy. It moves in sync with the broader canopy (I have no idea what this is supposed to mean). But it definitely sways. A second person always stands next to me (two is always better than one. So it is true in this dream). This person is usually well known to me. Sometimes they are not. In my dream, there is a tree limb that originates from the small platform. This tree limb is "totally occluded" (I know. Tree limbs in real life are always totally occluded. This one isn't supposed to be apparently). The goal is to cross and open this totally occluded tree limb. (I can't believe I am typing this for you to read.) The occluded limb traverses a great distance in the forest and connects to a separate platform in a separate tree often several hundred yards away from the base of operations platform. But the second platform is in the same forest. The goal is to get through the occluded tree limb: connect platform 1 with platform 2. The landing zone for the occluded limb is usually not visible in my dream. I need to rely on people on the second platform (there are always people on the second platform) to tell me if we were able to cross the occluded CTO tree limb. (I know, right? Weird.)

On the second platform is usually Grantham or Lombardi but not always. Using tree-sized CTO gear, I toil to connect the 2 distant trees through the aberrant wandering totally occluded tree limb. There is such clarity in this dream. The tools I use have surprisingly similar physical properties to the tools used in the CTO lab. (There is a tree-sized CrossBoss that spins easily from the platform in the occluded tree limb.) Sometimes I can get the gear to the second platform: the goal. Sometimes I cannot. When the going is difficult or slow, the team on the second platform sends gear to meet in the middle, also a goal in the dream. Somehow in the dream connecting in the middle of the tree trunk is also a success. Sometimes the folks on the second platform must leave their perch and trek across the forest ground and climb up to my platform to do it for me. (This makes Grantham grumpy sometimes. Yes. I know. I need more therapy. Can't make this up!) Sometimes I wake up before the platforms are connected. Sometimes people are watching and sometimes not. There are always 2 platforms. I am always high above the ground. Sometimes CTO tree limb crossing is easy, and sometimes it is hard. I don't know why this dream recurs, but I have come to believe this dream represents my perception that somewhere along the way I have become a capable CTO operator, which wasn't always the case, as you also know by now.

ADDITIONAL MISCELLANEOUS THOUGHTS
Practice Agency Often
You have the ability to use your voice, to use your words for a positive change. I think this is really important while you are working the lab and as a CTO operator. This comes in many forms. Probably the most important is to enable your cath lab team members to feel comfortable to exercise agency in the lab. They will notice things that you cannot. If they are empowered to speak and that when they do speak that they will effect positive change, your program and your practice and your patients will benefit. There are countless examples where astute cath lab team members improve outcomes when afforded this chance. But you need to do enough self-work to acknowledge that agency is important, and other agency is pivotal for your development.

You Are Still a Doctor
You are a CTO operator and a physician. Not long ago, and I really mean not long ago, a patient was referred to me in the office with a CTO of the RCA. She had a recent admission at a local hospital. She presented with shortness of breath and underwent a workup, which ended with a cardiac catheterization and the diagnosis of an RCA CTO. She had an ambiguous proximal cap with a higher-risk epicardial interventional collateral. As part of the decision making, I decided to get a coronary computed tomography (CT) angiography to better define her proximal cap. A week later, while she was still in the CT scanner, the radiologist called me to tell me she had a large saddle pulmonary embolus. Perfect. Great job! Don't forget you are still a doctor. Not all shortness of breath is a CTO of the RCA.

Unsuspecting Encouragement
You will receive encouragement when you least expect yet need it. You may, like me, receive it from unanticipated people. I received the most encouragement at one of my lowest points from a spouse of a patient who did not do well following CTO PCI. I failed to open his LAD, which meant that the transplant team would take over. Recall the institution didn't have much tolerance for reattempts at a failed procedure. As I was describing the failure to his wife, she was very calm and peaceful. She was centered and depressurized. She told me that she could sense that I was struggling. (I was in tears.) She encouraged me, as a woman of faith, to press on in what I believe in. She told me that she believed in me and in what we were trying to do. She encouraged me to continue to try to help other people like her husband. She shared with me that she believed I would succeed even when I was certain that I wouldn't. She gave me hope and strength and encouragement to press on. She believed in me when she had no reason to. She had faith when I did not. Without this conversation at this point in time, I am not certain how I would have navigated out of this very low valley. You will be encouraged when you need it.

I have elected to not cover the concepts of interoception and emotion management. But I should have. Please put this on your list of to do self-work.

SUMMARY

Last, I want to share with you sage advice given to me during trying times from close friends and counselors.

You are worthy. You are a worthy person. You are a worthy physician, friend, and colleague. Your value as a human, as a physician, as a friend, and as a colleague is not predicated on your success and failure rates. Your worth is not predicated on your complication rates. It is not based on how fast you are with retrograde CTO PCI or any other aspect of learning the CTO trade craft. You are worthy. Period.

Steven P. Marso, MD
Cardiovascular Service Line
HCA Midwest Health
Kansas City, MO 64132, USA

E-mail address:
Steve.Marso@HCAHealthcare.com

Indications and Patient Selection for Percutaneous Coronary Intervention of Chronic Total Occlusions

Taishi Hirai, MD[a],*, J. Aaron Grantham, MD[b,c]

KEYWORDS

- Chronic total occlusion • Percutaneous coronary intervention • Indications • Patient selection
- Angina • Quality of life

KEY POINTS

- Chronic total occlusion (CTO) percutaneous coronary intervention (PCI) should be offered to symptomatic patients with angina despite medical therapy, especially those with refractory angina (≥ 3 antianginal drugs).
- CTO operators should have a detailed discussion with the patient, prior to the procedure, outlining the projected risk and benefit of CTO PCI.
- Further studies are needed to clarify the role of CTO PCI in asymptomatic patients with low ejection fraction or asymptomatic ischemia.

INTRODUCTION

Chronic total occlusions (CTOs) are a commonly encountered complex coronary lesions, treated with profound variability that tends to be based on operator, not patient characteristics.[1] When CTOs are approached percutaneously, the vigor of the attempt might vary between operators from a "poke and hope" to "hail Mary" incredibly high-risk strategy that, in some cases, outweighs the potential for benefit. This article reviews the literature and discusses the indications for the procedure and how to appropriately select patients for CTO percutaneous coronary intervention (PCI) in hopes of inspiring the reader to more consistently offer this approach to indicated patients based on their symptoms, risk, and response to medical therapy, not the anatomy.

INDICATIONS

The most common indication for CTO PCI is angina relief, which translates into improved physical function and quality of life. Other, less-established indications include improvement of left ventricular (LV) function, reduction of ischemia, and complete revascularization, ostensibly for the purposes of improved survival in the absence of symptoms. Whether CTO PCI improves outcomes such as death and myocardial infarction is unknown and remains intensely debated.

Angina Relief

One of the major goals in therapy for patients with stable ischemic heart disease is the alleviation of lifestyle-limiting angina and angina-equivalent symptoms such as dyspnea and fatigue. Several observational studies have systematically used standardized, disease-specific, and prognostically important health status instruments such as the Seattle Angina Questionnaire (SAQ) and the Euro QOL-5D[2] to demonstrate significant improvements after successful versus unsuccessful CTO PCI.[3–5] The degree of baseline medical therapy, symptom

[a] University of Missouri, One Hospital Drive, Columbia, MO 65212, USA; [b] Saint Luke's Mid America Heart Institute, 4330 Wornall Road, Kansas City, MO 64111, USA; [c] University of Missouri-Kansas City, 2411 Holmes Street, Kansas City, MO 64108, USA
* Corresponding author.
E-mail address: hirait@health.missouri.edu

Intervent Cardiol Clin 10 (2021) 1–5
https://doi.org/10.1016/j.iccl.2020.09.002
2211-7458/21/© 2020 Elsevier Inc. All rights reserved.

burden, and selection bias confound these findings, but at very least these studies show expected outcomes in a real-world population selected for CTO PCI at predominantly high-volume CTO centers.

A recent, multicenter randomized control trial (the EURO-CTO trial) affirmed these benefits and extended the observations by finding greater improvement in SAQ scores among patients who underwent CTO PCI in addition to optimal medical therapy (OMT) compared to patients with OMT alone.[6]

It is important to note that to be included, patients had to have angina despite antianginal drug therapy with 2 agents. This should be the standard when selecting patients for CTO PCI. However, highly symptomatic patients were screened out from this study, which could underestimate the quality-of-life benefit of CTO PCI. Further, as in most PCI trials, enrollment was much slower than anticipated and represented only a small fraction of the cases performed at each center. In this regard, following the OPEN CTO study, a 12-center prospective study of patients undergoing CTO PCI, the authors' group reported that patients with refractory angina at baseline, defined as any angina despite 3 or more antianginal medications, have the largest quality-of-life benefit after successful CTO PCI ever reported (Fig. 1).[7]

Reduction of Ischemia
Historically, another goal of treatment for patients with stable ischemic heart disease was to simply reduce ischemia, regardless of symptoms, as ischemia was thought to be a valuable surrogate for prognosis.[8,9] In fact, these studies suggested that a reduction in ischemic burden of greater than 5% as assessed by myocardial perfusion imaging before and after revascularization was associated with improved survival. Another single-center observational study of patients undergoing CTO PCI reported that an ischemic burden of at least 12.5% is an optimal cut-off point that predicts greater than 5% reduction of ischemic burden after successful CTO PCI.[10]

The highly publicized ISCHEMIA trial, which randomized patients (including those with CTOs) who had moderate-to-high risk ischemia discovered by various forms of noninvasive tests to OMT and revascularization versus OMT alone prior to angiography, has been touted by many as proving this hypothesis to be false.[11] Although the study was beautifully designed, flaws in its execution have led some to question the validity of the results. For example, patient enrollment was much slower than anticipated, with very few enrollments per site relative to the procedural volume of these sites, suggesting the potential for selection bias or at least limiting the generalizability of the results to the entire population of patients with ischemia. The noninvasive studies were read and applied locally, prior to core laboratory adjudication, and the large proportion of moderate-to-high risk ischemia was based solely on treadmill exercise test findings. In addition, there was lack of imaging and angiographic correlation, lack of follow-up testing to confirm ischemia reduction, and poor completeness of revascularization (20% of the revascularization arm did not receive any revascularization). Because of these limitations, some cardiologists have deferred major practice

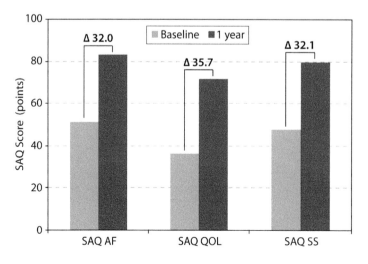

Fig. 1. Degree of improvement in quality of life in patients with refractory angina at 1-year follow-up compared with baseline assessed by Seattle Angina Questionnaire.

changes until additional data are reported for clarification.

Finally, specific to CTO PCI, it is important to note that most CTOs in the ISCHEMIA trial were not revascularized, and sometimes patients with CTOs (that were not revascularized) received PCI to nonischemic non-CTO vessel territories (David Maron and Philippe Genereux, TCT meeting, personal communication, October 2015). This practice was previously highlighted by Yeh and colleagues[12] in their courageous review of their practice before implementing a CTO PCI program.

The decision to offer a CTO PCI to a patient solely based on ischemia, in the absence of symptoms or LV dysfunction, remains controversial, and should be the focus of a shared decision-making exercise between patients and their care team in a comfortable office setting, not at the precatheterization preparation area or the postcatheterization recovery unit. What is not controversial, is that there is time to implement medical therapy and have these in depth discussions with patients and their families, as neither ISCHEMIA, nor other more CTO centric RCTs have shown any difference (either harm or benefit) in death or myocardial infarction (MI) with PCI to stable ischemic heart disease.

Improvement of Left Ventricular Function

Observational studies have reported improvement in LV ejection fraction (LVEF) after CTO recanalization.[13,14] However, these studies are limited by their nonrandomized design, where LVEF improvement could be confounded by other patient comorbidities and medical therapy.

The EXPLORE study was the first prospective randomized controlled trial to assess the effect of CTO PCI of nonculprit vessel on LVEF in patients presenting with ST elevation MI.[15] Although the overall results did not show a difference in the degree of LVEF improvement in patients who underwent CTO PCI compared with OMT alone, as assessed by cardiac MRI, a prespecified subgroup of patients with LAD CTO PCI had more improvement in LVEF compared with OMT alone. In another recent trial (the REVASC trial), CTO PCI was not associated with improvements in regional or global LV function. However, the mean baseline LV function was normal (>50%) in this study, precluding any conclusions about the association of CTO PCI with LV function improvement.[16] Therefore, further studies are necessary to study this population.

Complete Revascularization

Achieving complete revascularization is a major goal of treating patients with multivessel coronary artery disease. Previous post hoc studies suggested better outcomes with complete revascularization, assessed by the SYNTAX score, in patients with stable ischemic heart disease.[17] CTO is one of the main predictors of incomplete revascularization, and reported outcomes are worse with incomplete revascularization after CTO PCI.[18]

Reduction in Major Adverse Events

Studies have suggested that incidence of major adverse events was lower in patients who underwent successful CTO PCI compared with patients who underwent unsuccessful CTO PCI.[19,20] However, these studies were observational in design and thus limited by selection bias. The DECISION CTO study was designed to prospectively compare the long-term outcome in patients who underwent CTO PCI in addition to OMT with patients randomized to OMT alone.[21] However, because of numerous shortcomings such as slow enrollment, small number of cases per site, being underpowered, and high cross-over rates, the results have been inconclusive.

PATIENT SELECTION

As discussed previously, the primary indication for CTO PCI is reduction of angina. Before the procedure, it is important to have a detailed discussion with the patient, outlining the projected risks and benefits. At their institutions, the authors meet most patients in clinic before the CTO PCI, to go over symptoms and to discuss the treatment options. Moreover, when considering CTO PCI for less-proven indications such as improvement of LVEF or ischemia reduction, the authors will often discuss that these benefits are not validated by prospective randomized studies. It is the authors' practice to obtain viability testing such as cardiac MRI or positron emission tomography (PET) scan in those patients with low EF and to consider only patients with viable myocardium or with objective evidence of ischemia. Based on the previous studies, the authors often quote to their patients a risk of 6% to 7% of major complications and 85% to 90% procedural success rate.[22] The authors routinely discuss the possibility of a 2-staged procedure in the event of a failure. In this case, subintimal plaque modification (SPM) to facilitate flow through dissection planes can then improve success of repeat PCI attempts.[23,24] Patients and their families are an important part of the decision whether to proceed with CTO PCI.

On the other hand, it is also important for the operators to objectively assess their own skill level, equipment, and the experience of their catheterization laboratory staff when selecting these patients. For example, CTO PCI should not be performed in a hospital without surgical back up or by an operator of a catheterization laboratory team who would be unable to safely complete or bail out of a procedure should a complication occur. It is also appropriate for a relatively new operator to refer to a more experienced operator those higher-risk patients with challenging anatomy, such as need for use of epicardial collaterals.[25]

FUTURE DIRECTIONS

Future studies are needed in patient populations where the recommendation is unclear, such as patients with low EF without angina. Moreover, a study is needed that executes the intended design of the ISCHEMIA study by achieving complete revascularization by experienced CTO operators in the revascularization study arm. This would allow a true assessment of the effect of CTO PCI and complete revascularization. Finally, there is a need for prediction mechanisms, especially for less-experienced operators, to better assess the risk of complications, such as perforation. With these predictors, patients could be appropriately selected or referred to more experienced operators when necessary, which in turn could improve safety and efficacy for each patient undergoing CTO PCI.

CLINICS CARE POINTS

- CTO PCI should be offered to symptomatic patients with angina despite medial therapy, especially those with refractory angina (≥3 antianginal drugs).
- CTO operators should understand the current state of literature and have a detailed discussion with the patient about the risks and benefits of CTO PCI before the procedure.
- The risk-benefit calculation may be different depending on the experience of the operator.
- Further studies are needed to clarify the role of CTO PCI in asymptomatic patients with low EF or asymptomatic ischemia.

- A better prediction model of complications such as perforation would be useful for better patient selection.

DISCLOSURE

T. Hirai: honoraria from Abiomed. J.A. Grantham: speaking fees and honoraria from Boston Scientific, Abbott Vascular, and Asahi Intecc; institutional research grant support from Boston Scientific. He is a part-time employee of Corindus Vascular Robotics and owns equity in the company.

REFERENCES

1. Carlino M, Magri CJ, Uretsky BF, et al. Treatment of the chronic total occlusion: a call to action for the interventional community. Catheter Cardiovasc Interv 2015;85(5):771–8.
2. Brooks R. EuroQol: the current state of play. Health Policy 1996;37(1):53–72.
3. Grantham JA, Jones PG, Cannon L, et al. Quantifying the early health status benefits of successful chronic total occlusion recanalization: results from the FlowCardia's Approach to Chronic Total Occlusion Recanalization (FACTOR) Trial. Circ Cardiovasc Qual Outcomes 2010;3(3):284–90.
4. Borgia F, Viceconte N, Ali O, et al. Improved cardiac survival, freedom from MACE and angina-related quality of life after successful percutaneous recanalization of coronary artery chronic total occlusions. Int J Cardiol 2012;161(1):31–8.
5. Wijeysundera HC, Norris C, Fefer P, et al. Relationship between initial treatment strategy and quality of life in patients with coronary chronic total occlusions. Eurointervention 2014;9(10):1165–72.
6. Werner GS, Martin-Yuste V, Hildick-Smith D, et al. A randomized multicentre trial to compare revascularization with optimal medical therapy for the treatment of chronic total coronary occlusions. Eur Heart J 2018;39(26):2484–93.
7. Hirai T, Grantham JA, Sapontis J, et al. Quality of life changes after chronic total occlusion angioplasty in patients with baseline refractory angina. Circ Cardiovasc Interv 2019;12(3):e007558.
8. Shaw LJ, Berman DS, Maron DJ, et al. Optimal medical therapy with or without percutaneous coronary intervention to reduce ischemic burden: results from the Clinical Outcomes Utilizing Revascularization and Aggressive Drug Evaluation (COURAGE) trial nuclear substudy. Circulation 2008;117(10):1283–91.
9. Hachamovitch R, Hayes SW, Friedman JD, et al. Comparison of the short-term survival benefit associated with revascularization compared with medical therapy in patients with no prior coronary artery disease undergoing stress myocardial

perfusion single photon emission computed tomography. Circulation 2003;107(23):2900–7.

10. Safley DM, Koshy S, Grantham JA, et al. Changes in myocardial ischemic burden following percutaneous coronary intervention of chronic total occlusions. Catheter Cardiovasc Interv 2011;78(3):337–43.

11. Maron DJ, Hochman JS, Reynolds HR, et al. Initial invasive or conservative strategy for stable coronary disease. N Engl J Med 2020;382(15):1395–407.

12. Secemsky EA, Gallagher R, Harkness J, et al. Target vessel revascularization and territory of myocardial ischemia in patients with chronic total occlusions. J Am Coll Cardiol 2017;70(9):1196–7.

13. Galassi AR, Boukhris M, Toma A, et al. Percutaneous coronary intervention of chronic total occlusions in patients with low left ventricular ejection fraction. JACC Cardiovasc Interv 2017;10(21):2158–70.

14. Cheng AS, Selvanayagam JB, Jerosch-Herold M, et al. Percutaneous treatment of chronic total coronary occlusions improves regional hyperemic myocardial blood flow and contractility: insights from quantitative cardiovascular magnetic resonance imaging. JACC Cardiovasc Interv 2008;1(1):44–53.

15. Henriques JP, Hoebers LP, Ramunddal T, et al. Percutaneous intervention for concurrent chronic total occlusions in patients with STEMI: The EXPLORE Trial. J Am Coll Cardiol 2016;68(15):1622–32.

16. Mashayekhi K, Nuhrenberg TG, Toma A, et al. A randomized trial to assess regional left ventricular function after stent implantation in chronic total occlusion: the REVASC Trial. JACC Cardiovasc Interv 2018;11(19):1982–91.

17. Genereux P, Campos CM, Farooq V, et al. Validation of the SYNTAX revascularization index to quantify reasonable level of incomplete revascularization after percutaneous coronary intervention. Am J Cardiol 2015;116(2):174–86.

18. Azzalini L, Candilio L, Ojeda S, et al. Impact of incomplete revascularization on long-term outcomes following chronic total occlusion percutaneous coronary intervention. Am J Cardiol 2018;121(10):1138–48.

19. Yamamoto E, Natsuaki M, Morimoto T, et al. Long-term outcomes after percutaneous coronary intervention for chronic total occlusion (from the CREDO-Kyoto registry cohort-2). Am J Cardiol 2013;112(6):767–74.

20. Christopoulos G, Karmpaliotis D, Wyman MR, et al. Percutaneous intervention of circumflex chronic total occlusions is associated with worse procedural outcomes: insights from a multicentre US registry. Can J Cardiol 2014;30(12):1588–94.

21. Lee SW, Lee PH, Ahn JM, et al. Randomized trial evaluating percutaneous coronary intervention for the treatment of chronic total occlusion. Circulation 2019;139(14):1674–83.

22. Sapontis J, Salisbury AC, Yeh RW, et al. Early procedural and health status outcomes after chronic total occlusion angioplasty: a report from the OPEN-CTO Registry (Outcomes, Patient Health Status, and Efficiency iN Chronic Total Occlusion Hybrid Procedures). JACC Cardiovasc Interv 2017;10(15):1523–34.

23. Hirai T, Grantham JA, Sapontis J, et al. Impact of subintimal plaque modification procedures on health status after unsuccessful chronic total occlusion angioplasty. Catheter Cardiovasc Interv 2018;91(6):1035–42.

24. Hirai T, Grantham JA, Gosch KL, et al. Impact of subintimal or plaque modification on repeat chronic total occlusion angioplasty following an unsuccessful attempt. JACC Cardiovasc Interv 2020;13(8):1010–2.

25. Hirai T, Nicholson WJ, Sapontis J, et al. A detailed analysis of perforations during chronic total occlusion angioplasty. JACC Cardiovasc Interv 2019;12(19):1902–12.

Preprocedure Planning for Chronic Total Occlusion Percutaneous Coronary Intervention

The Separation Is in the Preparation

Allison B. Hall, MD[a,b,*]

KEYWORDS

• Chronic total occlusion • Preprocedural • Preparation • Strategy

KEY POINTS

• Successful execution of chronic total occlusion percutaneous coronary intervention is highly contingent on preprocedural preparation.
• Detailed preprocedural review of patient clinical traits and coronary anatomy is key to planning strategy and anticipating challenges.
• Developing a preprocedural approach to the intervention is crucial, with anticipation of intraprocedural challenges and familiarity with troubleshooting strategies and collection of equipment that is likely to be needed.
• Existing and potential safety concerns must be identified and properly prepared for.

INTRODUCTION

Successful chronic total occlusion (CTO) percutaneous coronary intervention (PCI) is achieved when the intervention has been technically successful and the procedure has been conducted as efficiently and as safely possible, avoiding intraprocedural complications or effectively managing those that ensue. There are no magic shortcuts to procuring the highest odds of achieving such success: the operator must devote adequate time to thorough preprocedural preparation. As the saying goes, even chance itself favors the prepared mind. Given the important role of preprocedural preparation, ad hoc CTO PCI is discouraged. Key aspects of preprocedural planning are outlined in this article.

PREPROCEDURAL PATIENT ENCOUNTER

Indication

Before proceeding with CTO PCI, both the operator and the patient must be entirely clear on why the procedure is being undertaken (Fig. 1). The benefits that the patient can reasonably be expected to gain through undergoing a successful intervention should be clearly delineated, as discussed elsewhere in this book with regard to patient selection. The appropriate indications for CTO PCI are outlined elsewhere in this issue. It is worth mentioning that avoidance of ad hoc CTO PCI and performing a detailed preprocedural patient assessment can also allow time to complete other helpful studies that might be needed in certain instances, such as an assessment of myocardial viability in the

---

[a] Eastern Health/Memorial University of Newfoundland, St. John's, Newfoundland, Canada; [b] C/O Cardiology Consultants, PO Box 23042, RPO Churchill Square, 8 Rowan Street, St. John's, Newfoundland A1B 4J9, Canada
* PO Box 23042, RPO Churchill Square, 8 Rowan Street, St. John's, Newfoundland A1B 4J9, Canada.
E-mail address: allisonhall7@gmail.com
Twitter: @A_B_Hall (A.B.H.)

Intervent Cardiol Clin 10 (2021) 7–23
https://doi.org/10.1016/j.iccl.2020.09.003
2211-7458/21/© 2020 Elsevier Inc. All rights reserved.

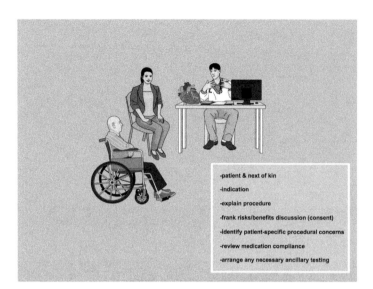

Fig. 1. The preprocedural encounter.

distribution of the vessel of interest, if this is in question.

Informed Consent

When possible, the patient should be accompanied by their next of kin during the consent process. The likelihood of technical success should be discussed with the patient and balanced with the potential risks. Contemporary series reflect technical success rates ranging generally between 85% and 90%, but include the range of hybrid algorithm strategies, and it is important for the CTO operator to consider their comfort with the demands of a particular case.[1] Patients must be fully informed about the potential intraprocedural and periprocedural risks of CTO PCI before agreeing to proceed and should understand that the risk is increased relative to non-CTO intervention.[2] Local experience can influence the numbers discussed, but many operators will quote an average risk of approximately 3% for serious complications.[1] The key potential risks to mention include coronary perforation with tamponade, vascular access complications, donor vessel injury, contrast-induced nephropathy, arrhythmias, radiation dermatitis, need for emergency coronary artery bypass grafting (CABG), or even death.[1,3] Last, it is imperative that the patient understand that CTO PCI carries the need for dual antiplatelet therapy, or an oral anticoagulation agent and P2Y12 inhibitor (if the former is otherwise indicated) and patients must understand the serious risk of noncompliance with same. If the patient does not value the

potential benefits over this realistic risk profile, then CTO PCI should not be pursued.

Anticipating Patient-Related Procedural Considerations

By meeting with a patient in advance of a CTO PCI, clinical traits specific to each individual can be recognized and planned for. Many different factors can be noted, of variable procedural significance. Importantly, for instance, if the patient has renal impairment, recognizing this factor in advance reinforces the use of intraprocedural strategies for contrast minimization, such as the use of preexisting imaging roadmaps, intravascular ultrasound-guided intervention, use of contrast-conserving systems such as DyeVert if available,[4] minimizing the number of injections, and sometimes preprocedural and postprocedural nephrologist consultation. If a patient is morbidly obese, this factor may increase the total radiation dose accumulation[5,6] and could impact procedural visualization or present vascular access challenges. If the patient has significant sleep-disordered breathing, this condition could be relevant for sedation protocols and some operators may choose to place the patient on continuous positive airway pressure or biphasic positive airway pressure during the case. Limb contractures or musculoskeletal complaints such as severe chronic back pain could require special positioning adjustments or additional sedation in order for the patient to tolerate a 2- to 3-hour procedure. The presence of peripheral arterial disease may present access issues, and may have higher in-hospital major adverse cardiac events and lower procedural success rates.[7]

STUDYING THE ANATOMY OF THE CHRONIC TOTAL OCCLUSION OF INTEREST

Participants

The operator(s) performing the CTO PCI (ie. interventional cardiologists, any participating fellows) must, of course, be involved in this aspect of preprocedural planning; however, especially in centers that do not have dedicated fellows or a second physician operator, consideration should always be given to including other members of the team such as nurses or techs so that they can become familiar with the anatomy of the case and the anticipated procedural strategies in advance (Figs. 2 and 3).

Dual Injection Angiography

CTO anatomy is best characterized by performing dual injection, with filling of the target vessel both in the antegrade fashion and in retrograde fashion from the donor vessel collaterals or bypass graft. Dual injection may at times be performed in advance during a diagnostic angiogram, with available films projected at the time of the CTO intervention, and this probably allows the most complete preprocedural planning;

typically, however, diagnostic angiograms with sufficient cine run to demonstrate collateral flow are sufficient to guide dual angiography views performed at the start of the CTO PCI case. If dual injection is performed during a diagnostic angiogram and there is desire to avoid adding an additional access point, it is possible to insert two 4F diagnostic catheters through a single 8F sheath, although this is not an optimal technique owing to worse visualization and catheter control.[3]

The injection should be performed with both vessels engaged with a guide catheter of adequate size to permit good vessel opacification. If 1 vessel is felt to be likely more difficult to engage than the other, it is best to engage the trickier vessel first, because the guide manipulation is unimpeded by the presence of a second guide. Some operators choose to engage a right coronary artery (RCA) first over a left main (LM) to avoid interacting with the guide sitting in the LM during RCA engagement.[3] Guides can be stabilized if needed by placement of a workhorse wire in the vessel of interest or in a neighboring branch, which also functions as a safety wire in the donor vessel. Many operators prefer to do this to aid urgent intervention in the event of donor vessel injury from the retrograde guide or equipment occurring during the PCI.

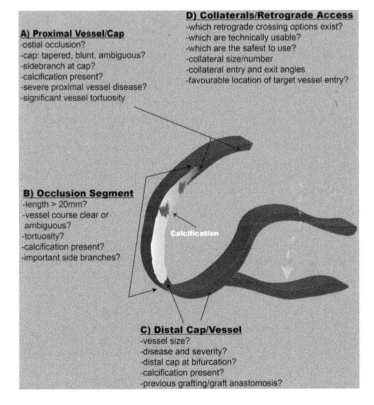

A) Proximal Vessel/Cap
-ostial occlusion?
-cap: tapered, blunt, ambiguous?
-sidebranch at cap?
-calcification present?
-severe proximal vessel disease?
-significant vessel tortuosity

D) Collaterals/Retrograde Access
-which retrograde crossing options exist?
-which are technically usable?
-which are the safest to use?
-collateral size/number
-collateral entry and exit angles
-favourable location of target vessel entry?

B) Occlusion Segment
-length > 20mm?
-vessel course clear or ambiguous?
-tortuosity?
-calcification present?
-important side branches?

Calcification

C) Distal Cap/Vessel
-vessel size?
-disease and severity?
-distal cap at bifurcation?
-calcification present?
-previous grafting/graft anastomosis?

Fig. 2. The 4 major angiographic components for detailed review from dual injection before CTO PCI.

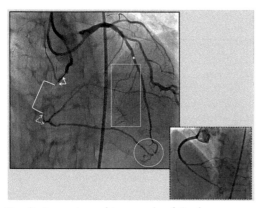

Fig. 3. An angiographic example of the four components for review from dual injection before a CTO PCI of the right coronary artery. *Solid arrows*, proximal vessel and proximal cap; *square bracket*, occlusion segment; *dotted arrows*, distal cap and distal vessel; *rectangle*, septal collateral channels; *circle*, tortuous epicardial channel. The proximal cap is tapered and there is no significant proximal vessel disease. The CTO segment is greater than 20 mm, but relatively unambiguous. The distal vessel is of relatively smaller caliber, but is not significantly diseased, though there is only a short segment before the distal RCA bifurcation. There are reasonable septal collaterals—small, but a relatively straight course and with direct connections; a less-favorable tortuous distal left anterior descending epicardial collateral is also present. The case was completed successfully with antegrade wire escalation (*dotted box*).

Dual injection images are best obtained at a low magnification and without panning.[3] Nitrate administration before injection may improve the visualization of the vessels and/or collaterals.[3] It is key to verify pressure waveforms before injecting, to ensure no catheter dampening is present that could result in vessel dissection upon injection. Side hole catheters waste some contrast into the aorta, but can be considered in instances such as RCA CTO PCI as an antegrade guide to avoid aortic dissection owing to pressure dampening. It can also be helpful to color code pressure tracings in a fashion that is easy to remember and to do it consistently from case to case-one option is to use red for the RCA and lime (green) or lemon (yellow) for the LM. Some operators engage the RCA through right-sided access points and the LM through left-sided access points as a memory aid, although each operator may have a different preference based on ergonomics, and so on; manifolds can be labeled as needed. The donor vessel is first injected to allow for adequate collateral filling of the distal CTO vessel and then the CTO vessel is injected shortly afterward. Certain angiographic projections will be more favorable for visualizing different types of collateral filling as is outlined in greater detail in Table 1.[3]

Of note, beyond injections for initial procedural planning, intraprocedural retrograde or dual injections are vital to accurately determining the position of wires and other equipment at various phases of the case. Performing a CTO PCI without dual visualization is a recipe for failure and complications.

Occasionally, a CTO will be encountered where only a single guide injection will permit antegrade and retrograde visualization of the target vessel when there is collateral supply only from ipsilateral vessels. A microcatheter can be used to better select the ipsilateral collateral to assist with visualization. This process is also helpful later in the case for selective retrograde injection so as to avoid antegrade injection and propagation of dissection or injury to the target vessel.[3] The ping-pong technique or the use of 2 catheters for entry to the same ostium, typically within the LM in left dominant systems, may be necessary for some ipsilateral collateral cases; this technique can help with retrograde equipment manipulation.[3]

Key Components to Examine on Dual Injection Angiography Images[1]

a. Proximal vessel and proximal cap
  - Is there an ostial occlusion? Ostial CTO PCI is particularly challenging and is among the instances where a retrograde approach is usually considered as the primary strategy.
  - Is the proximal cap ambiguous? If so, this may require preprocedural aids such as coronary computed tomography angiography (CCTA) as outlined further elsewhere in this article, the use of intracoronary imaging at the time of the procedure, or other specific strategies to resolve the ambiguity (Fig. 4).
  - Is the cap blunt or tapered/funnel-like? Tapered is more favorable for engaging the wire because this shape decreases ambiguity and aids in avoiding side-branch entry.
  - Is there a side-branch present at the proximal cap? This configuration can make directing the antegrade wire in the desired course toward the cap more challenging.
  - Is there heavy calcification of the proximal cap? This factor may make cap penetration more challenging and require the use of more penetrative wires or techniques to modify the proximal cap.

Table 1
Optimal angles for viewing various collateral connections

		Collateral Type	
	Septals	**Epicardial in Lateral Wall**	**Epicardial Between Proximal LCx and RCA**
Angulation	RAO Cranial → determining origin	LAO Cranial	AP Caudal
	RAO or RAO caudal → area closer to PDA	RAO Cranial	RAO
	LAO → may be helpful for wiring		

Abbreviations: AP, anteroposterior; LAO, left anterior oblique; LCx, left circumflex; RAO, right anterior oblique.
Data from Manual of Chronic Total Occlusion Interventions A Step-by-Step Approach by Emmanouil Brilakis, 2017.

- Is there severe disease in the vessel proximal to the proximal cap? This factor may impede wiring and may lead to guide catheter dampening and/or difficult equipment advancement.
- Is there severe tortuosity in the proximal segment? This configuration may necessitate enhanced guide support such as use of guide extensions or side-branch anchoring.

b. Occlusion segment
- What is the length of the occlusion? Longer occlusions, that is, greater than 20 mm, present more of a challenge than short occlusions, and this factor can potentially alter the crossing strategy.
- What is the course of the occluded segment? A straightforward and readily appreciated vessel course is more favorable, but highly tortuous segments or an ambiguous vessel course may present the need for further preprocedural imaging, early adoption of

retrograde wiring, or use of other means of resolving ambiguity. A tortuous segment will also generally make equipment advancement more difficult.
- Is there heavy calcification? This feature may cause challenging equipment advancement, can limit dissection–reentry zones/capability and may lead to the eventual need for plaque modification techniques and enhanced equipment support.
- Are there important side branches in the vicinity that could be lost depending on crossing strategy such as dissection–reentry?

c. Distal vessel and distal cap
- What is the size of the vessel? Successful crossing/reentry will be relatively easier in larger versus very small caliber vessels.
- Is the distal vessel severely diseased? This factor can hinder success in wire crossing

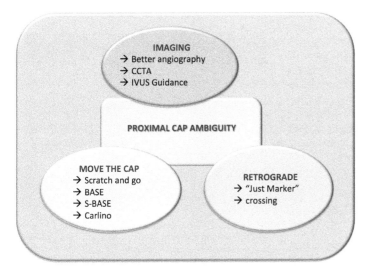

Fig. 4. Strategies for resolving proximal cap ambiguity. IVUS, intravascular ultrasound.

and reentry, and may favor a retrograde approach.

- Is the distal cap at a bifurcation? This will need to be factored into the crossing strategy (perhaps greater consideration of retrograde approach, potential dual lumen catheter use, etc) and may influence stenting strategy (bifurcation PCI).
- Is there heavy calcification? This factor can make wiring and intervention more challenging and can particularly hinder reentry if crossing from a subintimal plane.
- Grafted or nongrafted vessel? A nongrafted vessel's distal cap may be softer and more favorable for a retrograde crossing than might be the proximal cap exposed to higher pressure; however, a previously grafted vessel may have a distal cap with in fact more challenging penetration.[3] In addition, as wires cross and exit a CTO segment, occasionally they will pass into previous graft anastomoses in the distal vessel and recognizing the location and relationship of graft attachment sites to the CTO segment and distal vessel is very helpful for identifying and rectifying this phenomenon during the procedure. Cues include tenting of the vessel and subtle findings on fluoroscopy to demonstrate hinge points or calcification noted to run separately in some views.

d. Collaterals and retrograde crossing options
- Which retrograde crossing options are present? Retrograde crossing can be achieved via septal collaterals, epicardial collaterals, and via patent or occluded bypass grafts.
- Which collaterals are technically appealing in terms of feasibility of crossing? Collateral size and tortuosity are important predictors of crossability, with smaller and highly tortuous collaterals being harder to navigate.[3] Collateral size is graded according to the Werner classification[8] (Table 2). With respect to tortuosity, apart from acute angles within the collateral course, the angle of entry into the collateral vessel, as well as the angle of exit can influence success. Angles of greater than 90° help with entry more than acute angles.[3] As the wire enters the distal vessel, not only is the angle important, but the entry point should also be roughly greater than 10 mm from distal cap, or else it can be

harder to engage the cap.[3] Bifurcations or branch points along the course of collaterals can make wire passage harder as well. Finally, the number of collaterals present is worth noting; the greater the number, the more there are options and less chance of inducing ischemia, as can happen with crossing a solitary important collateral vessel. Collaterals can also be characterized by how well the distal epicardial vessel fills, the Rentrop classification[9] (Table 3).

- Among feasible options, which is likely to be the safest for the patient? As a general rule, in order of increasing risk, the following retrograde crossing conduits can be selected.[3]
  1. Bypass graft (non-left internal mammary artery [LIMA])
  2. Septal collateral
  3. Epicardial collateral
- Should the LIMA graft be used? Although it is technically possible and sometimes necessary to use a patent LIMA graft as retrograde access to a CTO, this technique is generally avoided unless absolutely necessary. The LIMA is very often a key remaining means of myocardial perfusion and any manipulation with wires and equipment across it can lead to transient but significant ischemia, either directly or through phenomena such as wire straightening its curvature, spasm of the vessel, or dissection with guide manipulation at often unfavorable angles. This strategy jeopardizes a potentially high-risk myocardial territory and thus use of the LIMA as a retrograde conduit

Table 2 Werner classification		
	Grade	Description
Included in original description	CC0	No continuous connection
	CC1	Thread-like continuous connection
	CC2	Side branch-like connection (≥0.4 mm)
	CC3	>1 mm diameter of direct connection

Data from Manual of Chronic Total Occlusion Interventions A Step-by-Step Approach by Emmanouil Brilakis, 2017.

Table 3
Rentrop classification

Grade	Description
0	No filling of collateral vessels
1	Filling of collateral vessels without any epicardial filling of target artery
2	Partial epicardial filling by collateral vessels of target artery
3	Complete epicardial filling by collateral vessels of target artery

Data from Manual of Chronic Total Occlusion Interventions A Step-by-Step Approach by Emmanouil Brilakis, 2017.

should be undertaken with caution by experienced operators.

- What if no or only faint or nonappealing collaterals are seen? Ensure good quality images have been obtained (ie, no panning, optimal angulation, breath hold as needed). Sometimes it may be necessary to perform a careful selective injection of a borderline collateral with a microcatheter engaged in the collateral to better delineate its course and to confirm the presence or lack of a connection.[3] If no obvious septal collaterals are noted on reviewing images, occasionally invisible connections can be successfully crossed with the use of the septal "surfing: technique intraprocedurally. If only a nonappealing epicardial collateral is noted, sometimes brief balloon occlusion across that collateral takeoff will lead to recruitment of otherwise not visualized septal collaterals.[3] Comparing current images with any available prior films of the occlusion can also help to identify collateral crossing options that may be present.
  - Review of non-CTO lesions of interest
    - Are there in fact other significant lesions in multiple territories that may indicate consideration of the option of CABG?
    - Are there any lesions proximal or distal to the CTO segment that may increase procedural difficulty?
    - If a retrograde approach is likely, does the donor vessel have any significant lesions that might require intervention to facilitate safe advancement of equipment? If so, it may be best to treat such lesions in

advance of the CTO PCI, or at the beginning of the procedure, if it is unlikely to excessively increase contrast or radiation use.[10]

- Scoring systems
  - CTO scoring systems offer a tool that can be used by the interventional cardiologist before CTO PCI to predict predominantly the level of anticipated difficulty and efficiency of the intervention and the relative likelihood of procedural success. The use of these scores, although longstanding, has recently become a matter of some debate in the CTO community; particularly in experienced centers, some practitioners believe that putting heavy consideration into more complex anatomic factors of a given CTO lesion (ie, higher score) may dissuade someone from offering revascularization to a patient who might otherwise serve to benefit and that anatomy itself should not dictate patient treatment over indication. However, the information resulting from CTO scoring systems can prove valuable for procedural planning in terms of predicting the complexity and duration of the case and, indeed, whether a given operator might best serve a patient by referring their case, if particularly complex, to a more experienced center. Using a combination of scores as well as reviewing the patient's symptom and clinical status in balance with lesion complexity and procedural risk can facilitate shared decision making with patients.
  - The most widely applied scoring system (with inception in 2011) is the Multicenter CTO Registry in Japan (J-CTO) score (**Fig. 5**), which predicts the likelihood of successful antegrade guidewire crossing within 30 minutes.[11] Many other scoring systems predicting various aspects of procedural success and other outcomes have been proposed and are listed:
    - In order of chronology of creation— many of these were previously summarized in a 2016 review by Karatasakis and colleagues[12]:
      - CL-Score,[13] Liu and colleagues[14] for predicting contrast-induce

nephropathy, Ito and colleagues,[15] Computed Tomography Registry of Chronic Total Occlusion Revascularization (CT-RECTOR) score (2015)

- PROGRESS-CTO score,[16] ORA score,[17] Chai and colleagues,[18] Wilson and colleagues[19] (2016)
- Ellis and colleagues,[20] RECHARGE registry score,[10] (2017)
- W-CTO score[21] (2018)
- EuroCTO Castle Score[22] (2019)

○ The purpose here is not to provide an exhaustive review of this multitude of scores, but rather to simply indicate them so that they can be further referenced by any operator as a part of the preprocedural planning process and with respect to the patient cohort that is most relevant to their case. It is perhaps worth briefly discussing the more recently conceived EuroCASTLE score (CASTLE = CABG history, ≥70 years of age, stump anatomy [blunt or invisible], tortuosity degree [severe or unseen], length of occlusion [≥20 mm], and extent of calcification [severe]), which was validated in the large EuroCTO registry.[22] When each parameter was assigned a value of 1, technical failure was seen to increase from 8% with a CASTLE score of 0 to 1, to 35% with a score of 4 or higher.[22] In a recent study, it was also found to be comparable to the J-CTO score in predicting CTO PCI outcome with a superior discriminatory capacity suggested for the more complex cases.[23]

- Also worth noting, is the incorporation into some scoring systems of CCTA imaging findings and the suggestion that this may improve predictive accuracy. The CT-RECTOR score makes use of CTA lesion characterization and when compared with the J-CTO Score, it provided more accurate prediction of efficient guidewire crossing and final procedural success.[24] In addition, when Fujino and colleagues[25] used CCTA parameters compared with use of conventional angiographic parameters to fulfill the J-CTO score

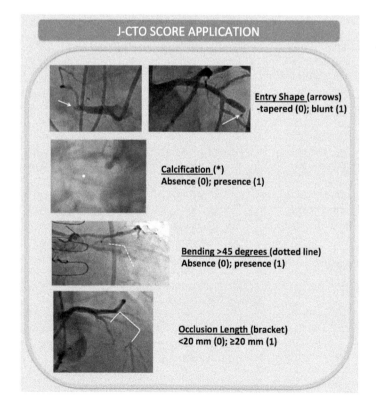

J-CTO SCORE APPLICATION

Entry Shape (arrows) -tapered (0); blunt (1)

Calcification (*) Absence (0); presence (1)

Bending >45 degrees (dotted line) Absence (0); presence (1)

Occlusion Length (bracket) <20 mm (0); ≥20 mm (1)

Fig. 5. Illustration of the components of the J-CTO score using angiographic examples.

in 205 consecutive patients who underwent CCTA before PCI, they found the CCTA version to be a more useful predictor of procedural success and 30-minute guidewire crossing. Further commentary on the value of CCTA in procedural planning is provided elsewhere in this article.

- Finally, the risk of periprocedural complications can be gauged using the PROGRESS-CTO complications score, comprised of 3 variables[26]:
  ○ Age ≥65 years (3 points)
    ○ Lesion length greater than 23 mm (2 points)
    ○ Use of the retrograde approach (1 point)
      ▪ ≥5 points: 6.6% risk of complications
      ▪ 3 to 4 points: 2% risk of complications
      ▪ 0 to 2 points: 0.2% risk of complications
- Use of adjunct imaging (CCTA)
- Sometimes, the course and characteristics of a CTO segment can remain unclear despite angiography. If available, and in collaboration with experienced imaging colleagues, CCTA can be extremely helpful to delineate a CTO in advance of undertaking PCI (Fig. 6). As noted in the scoring systems derived from these CT images, a CT scan can impart additional anatomic information that may be more accurate in certain cases than angiography alone. It can help to clarify an ambiguous cap, vessel tortuosity, and the length of the occlusion, and outline calcification. Anatomic clarification can be particularly useful by CT scan in patients with a history of redo CABG with multiple grafts to a single vessel.
- Importantly, where available, real-time CT fusion imaging is an emerging area in terms of anatomic information. CCTA images of a CTO vessel can be co-registered with fluoroscopic images at the time of the procedure and the use of such a "road map" could be very helpful, particularly in cases of ambiguous or tortuous vessel courses where wiring safety might be enhanced by this sort of guidance. The feasibility and potential implications of this CT fusion technique was showcased in a

study by Ghoshhajra and colleagues[27] that enrolled 24 patients who underwent CTO PCI using a prototype CT fusion software and who had a CT calcium and centerline overlay used intraprocedurally. This process was in comparison with 24 consecutive control CTO PCI patients without CT guidance.[27] Procedural outcomes and success were similar, but CT fusion added information regarding coronary arterial calcification and tortuosity that improved understanding in approaching antegrade wiring, antegrade dissection and reentry, and retrograde wiring during CTO PCI.[27] Further study in this area is warranted.

MAKING A GAME PLAN: CASE-SPECIFIC ORDER OF OPERATIONS

The final goal is successful CTO PCI; the question is how an individual operator feels he or she is most likely to safely and efficiently achieve this based on level of expertise and the traits of the case. CTO operators must plan how they intend to begin and progress through the procedure. Excellent algorithms exist to guide and inform decision making in terms of crossing strategies. A broad skillset will help to facilitate necessary and efficient maneuvering between strategies for ultimate success.

- Algorithms
  - The Hybrid algorithm,[28] which is represented (with the addition of subintimal plaque modification as a bailout option) in Fig. 7,[29] is a well-validated approach developed by North American operators, which was expanded upon with additional algorithms, including the Asia Pacific CTO Club algorithm[30] and the European CTO Club (EuroCTO) algorithm,[31] which incorporate consideration of further helpful components such as means of resolving proximal cap ambiguity (ie, intravascular ultrasound, BASE, scratch and go) and consideration of CrossBoss use for in-stent occlusions.[32] An additional algorithm was recently proposed by Tanaka and colleagues[33] that added focus on guidewire manipulation time and suggested a primary retrograde approach could be favored in cases

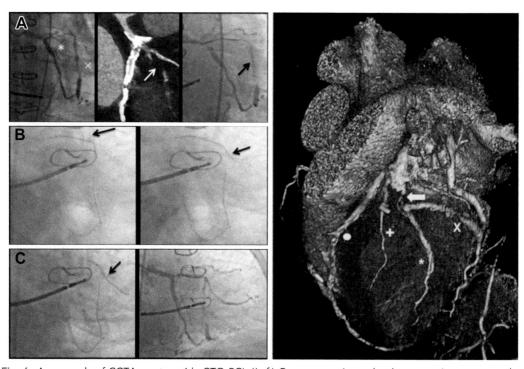

Fig. 6. An example of CCTA use to guide CTO PCI. (*Left*) Coronary angiography demonstrating near complete occlusion of a sequential saphenous vein graft (SVG) segment between the first and second obtuse marginal branches (OM1 and OM2) (*A, X*). The OM1 origin was unclear (*A, **). Emergency CCTA demonstrated that OM1 was actually the ramus branch that had a CTO (*A, white arrow*). Antegrade wire escalation attempts using a Corsair microcatheter and ultimately a Gaia Third guidewire, resulted in crossing into the SVG. sequential segment (*A, black arrow*). Using the dual operator, dual lumen microcatheter technique, a Sion Blue guidewire was advanced into the ramus (*B, C, black arrows*). After stenting antegrade flow was restored into the ramus (*C*). (*Right*) CCTA image, clarifying anatomy of the CTO vessel: what was described as a first obtuse marginal was a ramus intermedius branch (***). The CTO segment (*yellow arrow*), as well as the surrounding anatomy including a small branch off the ramus (*+*), the grafted left anterior descending artery (LAD) (*•*) and the diseased saphenous vein graft (SVG) skip portion (*x*) are delineated. CART, controlled antegrade and retrograde tracking; GFR, glomerular filtration rate. (*Reprinted from* Cardiovascular Revascularization Medicine, Vol 20, Hall AB et al, A Case-Based Illustration of a Dual-Operator, Dual Microcatheter Technique for Side Branch Wiring, Pages 21 to 25, Copyright (2019), with permission from Elsevier.)

where there was a CTO reattempt, when occlusion length was ≥20 mm and when there was no clear stump or visible entry antegradely into the occlusion, even with intravascular ultrasound. Guidewire manipulation time was shorter (107 vs 126 min) with primary retrograde over converted retrograde and it was felt that the need to convert to retrograde could be predicted by the aforementioned factors.[33] When the algorithm was retrospectively applied to the entirety of cases, more efficient and successful procedures were yielded if the algorithm was adhered to.[33] While this algorithm has generated interest and may prove useful, it has met with some criticism for various study limitations outlined in the accompanying review by Rinfret and colleagues,[32] which also nicely summarizes the aforementioned series of main algorithms.[34] One consideration was under-utilization of targeted antegrade dissection reentry (only 0.5% of the study population), a technique that is, well valued by many North American operators.[32] Realistically, the decision-making process is more nuanced given that a case may have variables that favor efficiency with an up-front retrograde approach according to the specifications of that algorithm/others, but it could be decided that a given

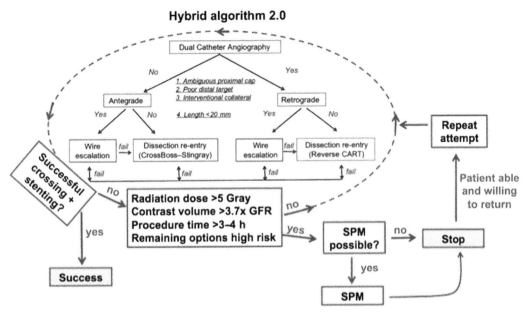

Fig. 7. Expanded hybrid algorithm incorporating subintimal plaque modification. (*From* Hall AB, Brilakis ES. Hybrid 2.0: Subintimal plaque modification for facilitation of future success in chronic total occlusion percutaneous coronary intervention. Catheterization and cardiovascular interventions: official journal of the Society for Cardiac Angiography & Interventions 2019;93:199-201; with permission.)

retrograde option could be relatively more high risk, making one inclined to still attempt antegrade first and to persist with it longer owing to relative danger.

- At the end of the day, at least across the aforementioned more well utilized and validated Hybrid-variety algorithms, a series of factors repeatedly arise that the operator can use to weigh decisions as to whether a retrograde solution is to be likely:
  - Blunt or absent cap/proximal ambiguity
  - Bifurcation at distal cap/poor distal vessel
  - Ostial vessel occlusion
  - Reattempt after unfavorable dissection extension during the initial attempt
- In contemporary practice, there is probably a general trend to at least briefly attempt an antegrade strategy first and it is unclear that factors such as the small amount of time saved with use of the algorithm developed by Tanaka and colleagues[33] will lead to shifts in practice over time. Ultimately, it is important to be flexible and to move between strategies, because persisting too long in either direction can be deleterious, such as creating a

burdensome large antegrade hematoma or attempting at length to navigate a highly tortuous epicardial collateral, only to perforate it.

- A recent consensus paper clearly outlines 4 key techniques for successfully crossing CTOs: antegrade wiring, antegrade dissection and reentry, retrograde wiring, and retrograde dissection and reentry.[1] Case examples of these are reviewed in detail in later sections of this issue. Familiarity with all of these techniques will increase ultimate success. Experience, along with the nuances of the various algorithms, will provide direction in each particular case as to how to navigate between strategies for the best outcome for the patient.
- Most of the algorithms include important safety criteria which should be factored into the decision to stop a procedure including[29,32]:
  - High contrast volume (>3.7–4.0× the estimated glomerular filtration rate)
  - High radiation exposure (air kerma >5 Gy and not well-advanced)
  - Potentially, procedure time greater than 3 hours if not well-advanced
- When the time is approaching to stop a CTO PCI based on safety criteria and

failure, bailout strategies or "investment" type techniques involving subintimal plaque modification such as subintimal tracking and reentry may be considered and, in fact, are included in the EuroCTO club algorithm.[31] Repeat angiography performed 2 to 4 months later, often shows lumen reconstitution/ dissection healing, and frequently, intervention can be completed with good likelihood of success and acceptable risk.[29,34]

Familiarity with Established Troubleshooting Strategies

In studying each CTO PCI case, one learns to anticipate particular challenges that might arise at various stages of the procedure. A multitude of potential obstacles may present themselves, particular to the anatomic and clinical traits of the case. Extremely helpful, "cookbook"-type approaches have been published or shared by experienced operators to help resolve the sorts of challenges that can arise in CTO PCI cases and it is worth being familiar with these algorithms well in advance so that they can be readily drawn upon during a difficult case for ultimate success. If a particular case is likely to cause any certain troubles more than others, it is worth refamiliarizing oneself with the algorithms for these issues before going into the procedure. Is there proximal cap ambiguity? Is there severe calcification that might make equipment advancement over the guidewire a challenge? Common challenges that can be encountered in CTO PCI are outlined in Box 1.[35] Just one example of an algorithmic approach for such problems is shown in Fig. 8 and many excellent resources exist for all challenges in sources, such as the *Manual of Chronic Total Occlusions Interventions*[3] or in the review paper entitled the "algorithms within the algorithms" by Riley and colleagues.[35]

Phone a Friend

Colleagues can be an invaluable resource when preparing for a CTO PCI. Particularly if a case is rather complex or a reattempt, it can be very helpful to review the films and approaches with an experienced operator beforehand. In certain instances of particularly challenging cases or early in one's experience, 2 CTO operators should participate directly. Finally, it is also key to consider referral onwards to a colleague/ different center as well, if one feels he or she

Box 1
Common challenges in CTO PCI: Know the algorithms
Wire impenetrable cap
Wire will cross the cap or lesion but gear will not follow
Proximal or distal cap ambiguity
Difficult anterograde dissection reentry
Wire across retrograde (bypass graft, septal or epicardial collateral) but microcatheter will not follow
Difficult retrograde dissection reentry
Cannot externalize wire during retrograde dissection reentry
Wire/gear keeps going into a side branch around/within a lesion
Difficult suture line to cross
In-stent CTOs
Data from Riley, RF et al, Algorithmic solutions to common problems encountered during chronic total occlusion angioplasty: The algorithms within the algorithm. Catheterization and cardiovascular interventions : official journal of the Society for Cardiac Angiography & Interventions 2019;93:286-297.

does not have the necessary skillset or equipment to safely and successfully proceed.

VASCULAR ACCESS

- The matter of selecting vascular access is detailed in another article in this issue, but in brief, it should be emphasized that planning the vascular access is a clear component of preprocedural preparation. At least 2, and rarely 3, access sites are desired for CTO PCI and which sites are available, safest. and also able to accommodate necessary equipment for the procedure must be determined in advance. In certain circumstances, patients may require vascular imaging studies to better inform the decision or, sometimes, intervention on vasculature in advance to permit access and equipment passage and this all must be sorted out before taking the patient for their CTO PCI. Planning vascular access may also require liaising with colleagues such as vascular surgery. As always, it should be ensured in advance that the equipment to facilitate safe vascular access such as ultrasound

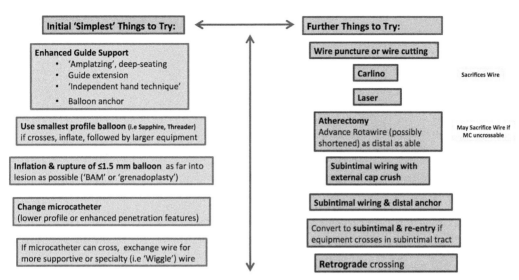

Fig. 8. An example of an algorithm: balloon or microcatheter uncrossable lesion. (*Data from* Riley RF, Walsh SJ, Kirtane AJ, Michael Wyman R, Nicholson WJ, Azzalini L, Spratt JC, Kalra S, Hanratty CG, Pershad A, DeMartini T, Karmpaliotis D, Lombardi WL, Aaron Grantham J. Algorithmic solutions to common problems encountered during chronic total occlusion angioplasty: The algorithms within the algorithm. Catheterization and cardiovascular interventions : official journal of the Society for Cardiac Angiography & Interventions 2019;93:286-297.)

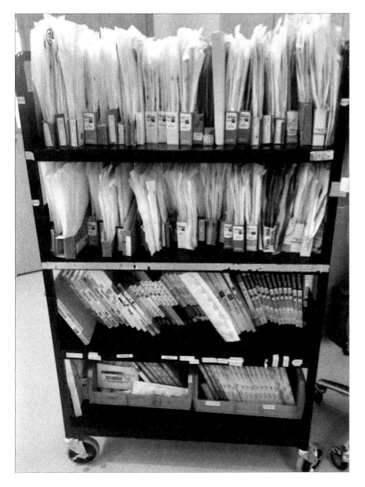

Fig. 9. An example of a CTO cart.

and micropuncture kits will be available at the time of the planned CTO PCI.

ANTICIPATING AND ENSURING AVAILABILITY OF NECESSARY EQUIPMENT

- Certain centers will have a plethora of CTO PCI equipment readily available, but for other centers this may not be the case. If there are limitations at play, the operator must ensure in advance of the procedure that all desired equipment will be present for the day of the case.

- One way to ease the burden of gathering necessary equipment preprocedurally and intraprocedurally, is to assemble a CTO cart at one's center that contains the majority of key equipment used during such cases (Fig. 9).

SAFETY PLANNING

- It is key to be well-trained and well-read in the algorithmic approaches to dealing with complications commonly encountered during CTO PCI. Next,

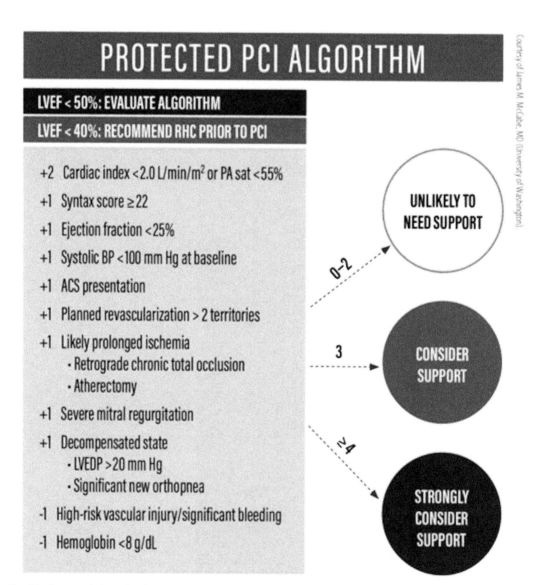

Fig. 10. Proposed algorithm for screening patients for protected PCI. BP, blood pressure; LVEDP, left ventricular end-diastolic pressure; PA sat, pulmonary artery saturation. (Courtesy of James M. McCabe, MD [University of Washington]).

having the potential equipment for complication management readily accessible, including for instance, intracoronary coils, covered stents, pericardiocentesis kit, is important. In some instances, if the case is particularly high risk, it may be worth involving additional operators or liaising with surgical colleagues on backup.

- Another component of safety planning is determining in advance whether the patient might benefit from up-front hemodynamic support or is at risk for potentially needing it. Again, this topic is outlined in greater detail in another article in this issue; however, the use of right heart catheterization and decision aids such as that shown in **Fig. 10**[36] can help to inform this decision. If one decides to use hemodynamic support up front, the device must be made available in advance, the downstream care of the patient arranged for and vascular access for the device prepared for.

- During the PCI, it will remain paramount to undertake strict radiation protection and reduction measures. Cine acquisition should be limited and the fluoroscopy store function can be used instead when possible. Low frame-rate fluoroscopy should be used, magnification and steep C-arm angulation should be avoided, and collimation and filters should be applied, with the image detector kept close to the patient.[37] Protective shielding and draping, along with personal protective equipment, should be maximized and real-time dose monitoring used if possible. Robot-assisted CTO intervention can be considered as an emerging area in capable facilities.[38]

- It will also be key to regularly check the activated clotting time throughout the procedure every 15 to 20 minutes to ensure it is kept in the range of 300 to 350 seconds (350 seconds for retrograde PCI) to decrease thrombotic complications.[3] Meticulous clearing and flushing of any equipment that looks suspect for thrombus or air during the procedure is also key. Always remember to clear the system of air after performing wire trapping.

- Donor vessel protection is also paramount and many operators may elect to place a safety wire in donor vessels for ready

treatment in case of emergency, such as vessel dissection. It is important to anticipate and account at all times for the effects of equipment manipulation on guide position and risk of vessel dissection.

SUMMARY

Potential additional considerations may arise in preprocedural planning for a given CTO PCI case, but if one takes all of these points into consideration consistently, this comprehensive procedural planning becomes more second nature for the operator for all cases, and he or she will truly recognize the separation in the ability to get through cases more smoothly and successfully.

DISCLOSURE

The author has nothing to disclose.

REFERENCES

1. Brilakis ES, Mashayekhi K, Tsuchikane E, et al. Guiding principles for chronic total occlusion percutaneous coronary intervention. Circulation 2019;140:420–33.
2. Brilakis ES, Banerjee S, Karmpaliotis D, et al. Procedural outcomes of chronic total occlusion percutaneous coronary intervention: a report from the NCDR (National Cardiovascular Data Registry). JACC Cardiovasc Interv 2015;8:245–53.
3. Brilakis ES. Manual of chronic total occlusion interventions a step-by-step approach. 2nd edition. Elsevier; 2017.
4. Tajti P, Xenogiannis I, Hall A, et al. Use of the Dye-vert system in chronic total occlusion percutaneous coronary intervention. J Invasive Cardiol 2019;31: 253–9.
5. Patterson C, Sapontis J, Nicholson WJ, et al. Impact of body mass index on outcome and health status after chronic total occlusion percutaneous coronary intervention: insights from the OPEN-CTO study. Catheter Cardiovasc Interv 2020. https://doi.org/10.1002/ccd.28928.
6. Yamamoto K, Sakakura K, Hamamoto K, et al. Determinants of Greater Peak radiation skin dose in percutaneous coronary intervention for chronic total occlusion. J Cardiol 2020;76(2):217–23.
7. Xenogiannis I, Gkargkoulas F, Karmpaliotis D, et al. The impact of peripheral artery disease in chronic total occlusion percutaneous coronary intervention (Insights From PROGRESS-CTO Registry). Angiology 2020;71:274–80.
8. Werner GS, Ferrari M, Heinke S, et al. Angiographic assessment of collateral connections in comparison

with invasively determined collateral function in chronic coronary occlusions. Circulation 2003;107: 1972–7.

9. Rentrop KP, Cohen M, Blanke H, et al. Changes in collateral channel filling immediately after controlled coronary artery occlusion by an angioplasty balloon in human subjects. J Am Coll Cardiol 1985;5:587–92.

10. Maeremans J, Spratt JC, Knaapen P, et al. Towards a contemporary, comprehensive scoring system for determining technical outcomes of hybrid percutaneous chronic total occlusion treatment: the RECHARGE score. Catheter Cardiovasc interv 2018;91:192–202.

11. Morino Y, Abe M, Morimoto T, et al. Predicting successful guidewire crossing through chronic total occlusion of native coronary lesions within 30 minutes: the J-CTO (Multicenter CTO Registry in Japan) score as a difficulty grading and time assessment tool. JACC Cardiovasc Interv 2011;4:213–21.

12. Karatasakis A, Danek BA, Brilakis ES. Scoring systems for chronic total occlusion percutaneous coronary intervention: if you fail to prepare you are preparing to fail. J Thorac Dis 2016;8:E1096–9.

13. Alessandrino G, Chevalier B, Lefevre T, et al. A clinical and angiographic scoring system to predict the probability of successful first-attempt percutaneous coronary intervention in patients with total chronic coronary occlusion. JACC Cardiovasc Interv 2015;8:1540–8.

14. Liu Y, Liu YH, Chen JY, et al. A simple preprocedural risk score for contrast-induced nephropathy among patients with chronic total occlusion undergoing percutaneous coronary intervention. Int J Cardiol 2015;180:69–71.

15. Opolski MP, Achenbach S, Schuhback A, et al. Coronary computed tomographic prediction rule for time-efficient guidewire crossing through chronic total occlusion: insights from the CT-RECTOR multicenter registry (Computed Tomography Registry of Chronic Total Occlusion Revascularization). JACC Cardiovasc Interv 2015;8:257–67.

16. Christopoulos G, Kandzari DE, Yeh RW, et al. Development and validation of a novel scoring system for predicting technical success of chronic total occlusion percutaneous coronary interventions: the PROGRESS CTO (Prospective Global Registry for the Study of Chronic Total Occlusion Intervention) Score. JACC Cardiovasc Interv 2016;9:1–9.

17. Galassi AR, Boukhris M, Azzarelli S, et al. Percutaneous coronary revascularization for chronic total occlusions: a novel predictive score of technical failure using advanced technologies. JACC Cardiovasc Interv 2016;9:911–22.

18. Chai WL, Agyekum F, Zhang B, et al. Clinical prediction score for successful retrograde procedure in chronic total occlusion percutaneous coronary intervention. Cardiology 2016;134:331–9.

19. Wilson WM, Walsh SJ, Yan AT, et al. Hybrid approach improves success of chronic total occlusion angioplasty. Heart 2016;102:1486–93.

20. Ellis SG, Burke MN, Murad MB, et al. Predictors of successful hybrid-approach chronic total coronary artery occlusion stenting: an improved model with novel correlates. JACC Cardiovasc Interv 2017;10: 1089–98.

21. Khanna RPC, Bedi S, Ashfaq F, et al. A weighted angiographic scoring model (W-CTO score) to predict success of antegrade wire crossing in chronic total occlusion: analysis from a single centre. AsiaIntervention 2018;4:18–25.

22. Szijgyarto Z, Rampat R, Werner GS, et al. Derivation and validation of a chronic total coronary occlusion intervention procedural success score from the 20,000-patient EuroCTO Registry: the EuroCTO (CASTLE) Score. JACC Cardiovasc Interv 2019;12: 335–42.

23. Kalogeropoulos AS, Alsanjari O, Keeble TR, et al. CASTLE score versus J-CTO score for the prediction of technical success in chronic total occlusion percutaneous revascularisation. EuroIntervention 2020;15:e1615–23.

24. Tan Y, Zhou J, Zhang W, et al. Comparison of CT-RECTOR and J-CTO scores to predict chronic total occlusion difficulty for percutaneous coronary intervention. Int J Cardiol 2017;235:169–75.

25. Fujino A, Otsuji S, Hasegawa K, et al. Accuracy of J-CTO score derived from computed tomography versus angiography to predict successful percutaneous coronary intervention. JACC Cardiovasc Imaging 2018;11:209–17.

26. Danek BA, Karatasakis A, Karmpaliotis D, et al. Development and validation of a scoring system for predicting periprocedural complications during percutaneous coronary interventions of chronic total occlusions: the prospective global registry for the study of chronic total occlusion intervention (PROGRESS CTO) Complications Score. J Am Heart Assoc 2016;5:e004272.

27. Ghoshhajra BB, Takx RAP, Stone LL, et al. Real-time fusion of coronary CT angiography with x-ray fluoroscopy during chronic total occlusion PCI. Eur Radiol 2017;27:2464–73.

28. Brilakis ES, Grantham JA, Rinfret S, et al. A percutaneous treatment algorithm for crossing coronary chronic total occlusions. JACC Cardiovasc Interv 2012;5:367–79.

29. Hall AB, Brilakis ES. Hybrid 2.0: subintimal plaque modification for facilitation of future success in chronic total occlusion percutaneous coronary intervention. Catheter Cardiovasc interv 2019;93:199–201.

30. Harding SA, Wu EB, Lo S, et al. A new algorithm for crossing chronic total occlusions from the Asia

Pacific Chronic Total Occlusion Club. JACC Cardiovasc Interv 2017;10:2135–43.

31. Galassi AR, Werner GS, Boukhris M, et al. Percutaneous recanalisation of chronic total occlusions: 2019 consensus document from the EuroCTO Club. EuroIntervention 2019;15:198–208.

32. Rinfret S, Harding SA. A new Japanese CTO algorithm: a step forward or backward? J Am Coll Cardiol 2019;74:2405–9.

33. Tanaka H, Tsuchikane E, Muramatsu T, et al. A novel algorithm for treating chronic total coronary artery occlusion. J Am Coll Cardiol 2019;74: 2392–404.

34. Xenogiannis I, Choi JW, Alaswad K, et al. Outcomes of subintimal plaque modification in chronic total occlusion percutaneous coronary intervention. Catheter Cardiovasc interv 2019. https://doi.org/ 10.1002/ccd.28614.

35. Riley RF, Walsh SJ, Kirtane AJ, et al. Algorithmic solutions to common problems encountered during chronic total occlusion angioplasty: the algorithms within the algorithm. Catheter Cardiovasc interv 2019;93:286–97.

36. Kearney K, McCabe JM, Riley RF. Hemodynamic Support for High-Risk PCI Patient selection and procedural strategy are key in treating this evolving patient population. Cardiac Interventions Today 2019;13:44–8.

37. Ison GR, Allahwala U, Weaver JC. Radiation management in coronary angiography: percutaneous coronary intervention for chronic total occlusion at the frontier. Heart Lung Circ 2019;28:1501–9.

38. Hirai T, Kearney K, Kataruka A, et al. Initial report of safety and procedure duration of robotic-assisted chronic total occlusion coronary intervention. Catheter Cardiovasc interv 2020;95:165–9.

Toolbox for Coronary Chronic Total Occlusion Percutaneous Coronary Intervention

Kathryn Dawson, MD, Amy Cheney, MD,
Ravi S. Hira, MD*

KEYWORDS

- Chronic total occlusion • Coronary guidewires • Microcatheters
- Antegrade dissection and reentry

KEY POINTS

- With development of new devices for CTO PCI it is important to categorize them broadly by design and intended task.
- This enables a safe and systematic approach to CTO PCI and avoid overlap and waste.
- Multiple options for coronary guidewires, microcatheters, balloons, snares, guide extensions, and tools for complication management are discussed.

INTRODUCTION

Since the publication of the hybrid algorithm, the toolbox for coronary chronic total occlusion (CTO) percutaneous coronary intervention (PCI) has continued to expand with rapid development of new specialty wires, microcatheters, guide extensions, lower profile balloons, and use of intracoronary imaging and hemodynamic support to facilitate successful antegrade and retrograde CTO PCI.[1] With the development of new devices, it is important to categorize them broadly by design and intended tasks. This would avoid adding inventory that is similar to that already on the shelf and prevent overlap and waste.

This article serves as a guide for tool selection for the interventional cardiologist performing CTO PCI. We discuss specialty guidewires, microcatheters, guide extensions, dedicated antegrade dissection and reentry devices, specialty balloons, snares, use of intracoronary imaging modalities, devices for calcified vessels, and tools for complication management and their role in CTO PCI.

CORONARY GUIDEWIRES

Coronary guidewires have a wide array of available options for the interventional operator, for routine PCI and more complex coronary interventions. Many coronary guidewires have similar technical design and can serve similar functions during coronary interventions, which makes wire selection a challenging task for operators. An operator does not need access to all of the commercially available wires to perform successful CTO intervention. Instead, many operators advocate for having a few "must-have" wire types designed to tackle specific tasks. This section serves as a reference for the types of coronary guidewires typically used during CTO PCI.

Coronary guidewires can generally be divided into polymer jacketed versus nonjacketed wires.

Department of Cardiology, University of Washington Medical Center, 1959 NE Pacific Street, Box 356422, Seattle, WA 98195, USA
* Corresponding author. 325 Ninth Avenue, Box 359748, Seattle, WA 98104.
E-mail address: hira.ravi@gmail.com

Intervent Cardiol Clin 10 (2021) 25–31
https://doi.org/10.1016/j.iccl.2020.09.011
2211-7458/21/© 2020 Elsevier Inc. All rights reserved.

Nonjacketed wires provide more tactile feedback to avoid unintended dissections and perforations. Polymer jacketed wires reduce friction often allowing for easier passage through small channels and in the subintimal space but at the cost of reduced tactile feedback. Wires are further differentiated by whether they have a tapered tip, which increases the penetration force of the wire, or a nontapered tip.[2]

For CTO procedures, wires are categorized based on the specific task or function they serve during the procedure. Some of the most commonly used wires for CTO PCI are listed in Table 1 and categorized by function.

Penetration Wires

Penetration wires are a spectrum of stiff wires ranging from the Fielder XT (Asahi Intecc, Seto-Shi, Japan) at the lower end to an Astato 8-20 (Asahi Intecc) at the higher end. As stiffness, tip force, and penetration power increase, the potential for such complications as vessel perforation also increase. Therefore, most operators recommend using these wires in a graded fashion during antegrade or retrograde wire escalation. The primary function served by these wires is to penetrate the proximal (when approached antegrade) or distal cap (when approached retrograde) and in some instances to scratch into the subintimal space. Once this has been done, rapid de-escalation to a less stiff wire is recommended. The stiff penetration wire should not be used to cross the entire length of the CTO segment, especially if it is greater than 20 mm in length when dissection reentry techniques should be used instead. Because of their high penetration power these wires are also commonly used in Stingray-based antegrade dissection and reentry techniques to puncture into the distal true lumen from the subintimal space.[3]

Knuckle/Dissection Wires

Once access has been obtained to the subintimal space at the proximal or distal cap, stiff, polymer jacketed wires, such as the Gladius Mongo wire (Asahi Intecc) and the Fielder XT family of wires (Asahi Intecc) are used for knuckling around the CTO lesion in the subintimal space.[4] This is because they tend to form smaller knuckles that create less subintimal hematoma and still provide information regarding vessel size, branch vessel, or perforation based on the size of the knuckle they form. Wires from the first-line penetration wire category, such as the Pilot 200 (Asahi Intecc), Gladius (Asahi Intecc), and Raider (Teleflex, Wayne, PA) coronary guidewires, can also be used for knuckling; however, because of their stiffness they tend to form larger knuckles and are considered second line for knuckling. These larger knuckles are used to avoid smaller branch vessels but come with the disadvantage of a larger dissection plane and larger subintimal hematoma making reentry challenging. Fig. 1 demonstrates the common wire shapes that are formed in CTO PCI.

Table 1
Coronary guidewire options based on wire characteristics and function

Wire Function	Wire Characteristics	Wires	Tip Stiffness (g)	Manufacturer
First-line penetration wires	Polymer jacketed	Pilot 200	4.1	Asahi Intecc
		Gladius	3.0	Asahi Intecc
		Raider	3.0	Teleflex
Second-line penetration wires	Nonjacketed	Confianza Pro 12	12.4	Asahi Intecc
		Hornet 14	14	Asahi Intecc
		Astato 8-20	8-20	Boston Scientific
		Gaia 1, 2, 3, Next	1.7, 3.5, 4.5	Asahi Intecc
Knuckling wires	Polymer jacketed	Gladius Mongo	3.0	Asahi Intecc
	Polymer jacketed wire	Fielder XT,	0.8, 1.0	Asahi Intecc
	Tapered tip	XT-A Fighter	1.5	Boston Scientific
Collateral wires for retrograde crossing	Nonjacketed Polymer jacketed	Sion	0.7	Asahi Intecc
		Suoh3	0.3	Asahi Intecc
		Samurai RC	1.2	Boston Scientific
		Fielder FC, XT-R	0.8, 0.6	Asahi Intecc
		Sion Black	0.9	Asahi Intecc
Externalization wires	Hydrophilic coating	R350	3.0	Teleflex
		RG3	3.0	Asahi Intecc

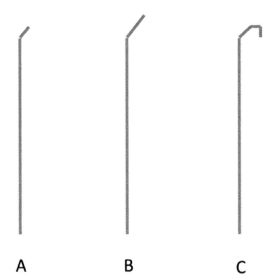

A   B   C

Fig. 1. Wire tip shapes used in CTO PCI. (*A*) Wire shape to penetrate a proximal or distal cap. (*B*) Longer wire tip to facilitate scratching into the subintimal space or performing reverse controlled antegrade and retrograde tracking (CART). (*C*) Wire shaped for knuckling in dissection and reentry. The "umbrella hook" shape.

Collateral Crossing Wires

For retrograde and collateral wiring techniques, wires with low tip stiffness, good torquability, and flexible shafts are ideal to traverse the septal and epicardial tortuous channels while limiting unintended wire perforation. These include the Sion, Suoh3, and the Sion Black (Asahi Intecc) and the Fielder FC, Fielder XT-R (Asahi Intecc), and Samurai RC (Boston Scientific, Marlborough, MA).

Externalization Wires

These wires are more than 330 cm in length and have a hydrophilic coating on the body of the wire facilitating externalization in retrograde techniques. Once the retrograde crossing wire or penetration wire has been advanced along with the microcatheter through the collateral into the antegrade guide, the short wire is removed and the externalization wire is then advanced. This is done such that the tip of the externalization wire is introduced through the retrograde microcatheter and guide, advanced through the collateral, up the target vessel, and into and out of the antegrade guide. This provides control of both ends of the wire. Devices can then be advanced antegrade over the soft tip of this wire to perform PCI. The R350 (Asahi Intecc) and the RG3 (Vascular Solutions, Charlotte, NC) are the most commonly used externalization wires. We routinely use the

R350, which is a 350-cm wire with a nitinol core and is kink resistant, whereas the RG3 has a stainless-steel core making it more prone to kinking.

MICROCATHETERS

Microcatheters are routinely used during CTO PCI to provide additional support for the guidewire and thereby increase the penetration power. They also facilitate rapid wire exchange and reshaping once the base of operations has been advanced. In addition to their support and exchange purposes, microcatheters are used to dilate channels, facilitate intracoronary drug delivery, and to perform localized contrast injections.[5] Some operators use over-the-wire balloons for added penetration force rather than a microcatheter, but microcatheters are generally preferred because they are more deliverable through tortuous segments and are less prone to kinking. There are now many commercially available microcatheters with different crossing profiles, torquability, deliverability, and lengths. Longer 150-cm catheters are needed for retrograde interventions.

The Caravel (Asahi Intecc), Finecross (Terumo, Shibuya, Japan), and Micro-14 (Roxwood Medical, Redwood City, CA) microcatheters are similar in that they are very-low-profile catheters that are useful for navigating very small channels that the larger microcatheters may have trouble traversing. However, because of their design, they have limited torque transmission and pushability.[4,6] The larger microcatheters, such as the Corsair family of microcatheters and the Turnpike family of microcatheters, provide improved support through calcified segments and better torque transmission than the smaller microcatheters. The Turnpike LP (Teleflex), Mamba Flex (Boston Scientific), and Corsair Pro XS (Asahi Intecc) are smaller profile than the other catheters within the Turnpike and Corsair families and are designed to facilitate retrograde crossing. The Turnpike Gold and Tornus microcatheters have stiffer tips and are useful for dottering vessels when other microcatheters do not cross. It should be noted, however, that the Tornus microcatheter does not have an inner polymer lining and as such cannot be used for injection of contrast (Table 2).

DUAL-LUMEN MICROCATHETERS

Dual-lumen microcatheters are comprised of a rapid exchange segment at the distal end of the catheter and an over-the-wire segment

Table 2
Commonly used microcatheters listed in order of crossing profile

Microcatheter	Length	Distal Shaft (French Catheter)	Manufacturer
Micro-14	155 cm	1.6	Roxwood Medical
Finecross	130 cm, 150 cm	1.8	Terumo
Caravel	135 cm, 150 cm	1.9	Asahi Intecc
Corsair Pro XS	135 cm, 150 cm	2.1	Asahi Intecc
Mamba Flex	135 cm, 150 cm	2.1	Boston Scientific
Turnpike LP	135 cm, 150 cm	2.2	Vascular Solutions
Mamba	135 cm	2.3	Boston Scientific
Corsair	135 cm, 150 cm	2.6	Asahi Intecc
Corsair Pro	135 cm, 150 cm	2.6	Asahi Intecc
Tornus	135 cm	2.1, 2.6	Asahi Intecc
Turnpike	135 cm, 150 cm	2.6	Vascular Solutions
Turnpike Spiral	130 cm, 150 cm	2.9	Vascular Solutions
Turnpike Gold	135 cm	2.9	Vascular Solutions

proximally that extends the entire length of the catheter. Dual-lumen catheters are used for a variety of purposes including side branch wiring in CTO and non-CTO PCI. Notably, they can also be used as tools for drug delivery or contrast injection in the distal vessel through the over-the-wire portion of the catheter. The two commercially available dual-lumen catheters available in the United States are the Twin Pass (Vascular Solutions) and the Sasuke (Asahi Intecc). The Sasuke has a smaller crossing profile.

GUIDE EXTENSIONS

Successful complex coronary interventions often require additional guide support for successful delivery of interventional gear to the distal vessel. There are several commercially available guide extensions that come in a range of sizes depending on the size of the guide catheter used. The most commonly used guide extensions range from 6F to 8F catheter. An additional guide extension that is specifically designed for CTO PCI is the Trapliner (Teleflex), which combines a rapid exchange guide extension catheter and trapping balloon.

Having the ability to rapidly exchange out gear while maintaining wire position is useful for improving efficiency during complex interventions. Guide extensions can also be used to plug the inflow of blood into the subintimal space to prevent subintimal hematoma expansion when performing antegrade dissection

reentry. The Trapliner is uniquely helpful for this because the trapping balloon enables exchanges of the microcatheter, Crossboss (Boston Scientific), and Stingray balloon (Boston Scientific) in a 6F catheter system.

ANTEGRADE DISSECTION REENTRY DEVICES

Step-by-step antegrade dissection and reentry techniques are discussed elsewhere in this issue. In brief, it is a technique that facilitates traversing around the CTO segment in the subintimal space and performing targeted reentry back into the true lumen distal to the CTO segment. This is usually performed in lesions that are greater than 20 mm with a clearly defined proximal cap and a good distal reentry target.[1] The equipment specifically designed for this purpose is the Crossboss catheter and Stingray Balloon System (Boston Scientific).

The Crossboss is a metal-braided, over-the-wire support catheter with a blunt atraumatic 1-mm tip that is advanced easily in the subintimal space using a fast-spin technique (Fig. 2A).[7] It is designed to create a controlled dissection in the subintimal space that helps facilitate delivery of the Stingray balloon while minimizing the subintimal hematoma.[8] The Crossboss catheter can also be particularly useful when crossing true lumen to true lumen for in-stent CTO because the stent struts prevent the catheter from exiting the stent.[3]

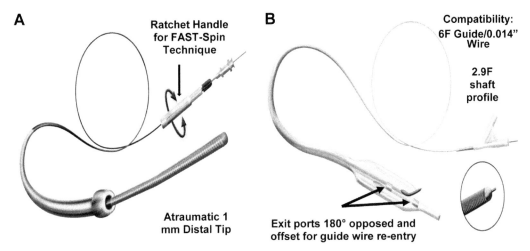

Fig. 2. (*A*) The Crossboss catheter, a 0.014-inch guidewire-compatible over-the-wire catheter with a 1-mm blunt tip. (*B*) Stingray balloon and guidewire. (Image provided courtesy of Boston Scientific. ©2020 Boston Scientific Corporation or its affiliates. All rights reserved.)

The Stingray balloon catheter and guidewire system is comprised of a flat, low-profile, over-the-wire balloon with two exit ports and a stiff guidewire that has a tapered tip and a distal probe. Once the Crossboss catheter has been used to cross around the CTO segment in the subintimal space, the Stingray balloon and guidewire is used to reenter into the distal true lumen in a targeted fashion. The Stingray balloon has a flat shape when inflated at low pressure (3–4 atm) with three exit ports. One is the distal over-the-wire exit port, and the other two exit ports are 180° opposed and offset for selective guidewire puncture and entry into the true lumen (**Fig. 2**B). We routinely use a Miracle Bros 12 wire to deliver the Stingray balloon because of its stiffness extending through the body to the wire tip. We use the Confianza Pro 12, Hornet 14, or Astato 8-20 for puncturing out the exit ports instead of the Stingray wire and the Pilot 200 or Gladius when swapping for a wire to advance in the distal true lumen.

BALLOONS

A common mode of failure encountered in CTO PCI is an inability to deliver microcatheters and devices across the lesion once the wire is across it. If the use of additional guide support with a guide extension is unsuccessful the microcatheter is exchanged out for a small, semicompliant balloon (1.0, 1.25, or 1.5 × 20 mm). Serial inflations are then performed to pass the balloon across the lesion. If successful, the balloon is exchanged out for a microcatheter. We routinely use small-diameter balloons in this scenario because these balloons have only one radiopaque marker in the center of the balloon as compared with balloons that are greater than 2 mm in diameter that have two radiopaque markers at each end of the balloon. The markers are usually the thickest part of the balloon and therefore, small-diameter balloons facilitate better crossing and delivery further into the occlusive segment.[3]

Long 40-mm balloons can also be useful, particularly during balloon angioplasty in the subintimal space. In addition to decreasing fluoroscopy time by reducing the number of required inflations, long balloons can reduce the risk of perforation by distributing the inflation pressure over a longer length, as opposed to shorter balloons, which concentrate pressure over shorter distances and focal lesions.

SNARES

When the retrograde wire cannot be directed into the antegrade guide a snare may be needed to successfully externalize the retrograde wire. The three-loop (tulip shaped) snares are typically more effective at capturing a guidewire than single-loop snares, although both can be used. Most fit through a 6F catheter guide, although some of the larger tulip-shaped snares require a 7F catheter guide. Of note, one should always snare a long (300-cm wire or longer) wire because of risk of losing control of the wire or entrapment.

INTRAVASCULAR IMAGING

Intravascular imaging has become a crucial part of routine and complex coronary interventions.

Benefits include understanding plaque morphology and calcification that may require additional vessel preparation with atherectomy and stent sizing and optimization to prevent future stent failure and restenosis.[9] It has also been demonstrated to be useful in CTO, with the 2-year follow-up of the AIR-CTO trial demonstrating lower rates of late lumen loss when compared with angiography-guided CTO interventions.[10]

In addition to improving clinical outcomes, intravascular imaging is increasingly used to achieve successful wire crossing in CTO PCI, by resolving proximal cap ambiguity and by facilitating challenging reverse CART scenarios. The role of intravascular imaging in CTOs and techniques for improving the success rate and durability of CTO PCI are discussed elsewhere in this issue. Briefly, the two primary modalities for intracoronary imaging are intravascular ultrasound (IVUS) and optical coherence tomography. In the United States the IVUS catheters available are the Opticross catheter (Boston Scientific), the Eagle Eye Platinum, and Eagle Eye Platinum ST (Philips, Eindhoven, the Netherlands). The Eagle Eye Platinum ST catheter has a shorter tip to imaging distance and as such is more deliverable when trying to image the proximal cap. The Opticross HD catheter (Boston Scientific) has higher image resolution, which can improve characterization of plaque morphology and is a 5F catheter system, but is challenging to deliver to the imaging segment.

Under most circumstances, optical coherence tomography (Abbott Vascular) provides higher image resolution in the near field. However, because of the need for high osmolality medium to clear the vessel for imaging, image resolution during CTO intervention is limited because of poor outflow of the segment. Additionally, because CTO PCI often requires purposeful dissection into the subintimal space, antegrade injections are specifically avoided in most cases to avoid distal hydraulic dissection propagation. For these reasons IVUS is often our preferred imaging modality in CTO interventions.

MANAGEMENT OF CALCIFICATION

Chronically occluded vessels and complex coronary lesions are frequently accompanied with heavy calcification making additional tools for plaque modification an important aspect of any interventional operator's toolbox. This section discusses the use of atherectomy in CTO PCI and a newer calcium modification technology.

Atherectomy

The indications, device specifications, and step-by-step instructions for atherectomy are beyond the scope of this article. For lesions that require additional plaque modification, rotational atherectomy (Boston Scientific) is our preferred atherectomy device for use in CTO. Because many CTO interventions require working in the subintimal space, we recommend no larger than a 1.5 burr to limit the risk of perforation or stalled burrs while working in a dissection plane. For this same reason orbital atherectomy (Cardiovascular Solutions, Inc) is avoided within the subintimal plane because the mechanism of action of orbital atherectomy can cause the catheter to propagate the dissection. Finally, we primarily use laser atherectomy (Philips) for in-stent restenosis and to soften the proximal cap in uncrossable lesions.

Shockwave Lithoplasty

Although still off-label for coronary calcium modification in the United States, intracoronary lithoplasty or Shockwave (Shockwave Medical, Santa Clara, CA) has been gaining popularity for modification of circumferential calcium in Europe. In regard to its use in CTO PCI, it will likely be most useful within the true lumen of the vessel when there is a greater than 270° arc of calcium on intravascular imaging. In segments across the subintimal space the adventitia comprises one side of the new lumen and thus lithoplasty is of limited utility even for undilatable lesions.

TOOLS FOR COMPLICATION MANAGEMENT

Risk factors and management for complications during CTO PCI are discussed elsewhere in this issue. Mechanical support options during PCI as an upfront strategy for high-risk cases and in emergent situations with hemodynamic collapse are also discussed elsewhere in this issue.

Management of coronary perforations and tamponade requires that CTO operators are facile with rapid access to the pericardial space for emergent pericardiocentesis when required. Embolization is done with the use of thrombin or fat injections or with the use of coil embolization devices. Operators should be well versed with the steps for coil embolization and which coils and catheters are compatible to deliver them to the site of perforation.

Covered stents are also an important tool that should be available in any catheterization laboratory performing complex PCI for use when conservative measures, such as balloon tamponade and pericardiocentesis, are ineffective. Previously the only available covered stent was the Jostent Graftmaster (Abbott Vascular), which had graft material sandwiched between two stainless-steel stents. Sizes ranged from 2.8 to 4.0 mm, which required a 6F catheter guide to 4.5 to 4.8 mm, which required a 7F catheter guide. Regardless of the size, the Graftmaster was challenging to deliver because of its large crossing profile. More recently the PK Papyrus covered stent (Biotronik, Berlin, Germany) is available, which has a single layer of stent resulting in a lower crossing profile and improved deliverability. A chart comparing the technical design of the Jostent Graftmaster with the PK Papyrus stent is seen here: http://www.biotronik. com/en-us/products/vi/coronary/pk-papyrus.

SUMMARY

CTO PCI has continued to evolve with increased uptake and implementation of antegrade and retrograde techniques among operators. This has resulted in the development of a wide variety of tools available to the operator. Although a few specific tools are required to ensure safe and successful CTO PCI, it is important to categorize devices with a functional purview so the entire team is well-versed in the pros and cons of each device and facilitates a safe and systematic approach to CTO PCI while avoiding overlap and optimizing resource utilization.

DISCLOSURE

Dr R.S. Hira consults for ASAHI Intecc and Abbott Vascular Inc.

REFERENCES

1. Brilakis ES, Grantham JA, Rinfret S, et al. A percutaneous treatment algorithm for crossing coronary chronic total occlusions. JACC Cardiovasc Interv 2012;5(4):367–79.
2. Creaney C, Walsh SJ. Antegrade chronic total occlusion strategies: a technical focus for 2020. Interv Cardiol Rev 2020;15:e08.
3. Riley RF, Walsh SJ, Kirtane AJ, et al. Algorithmic solutions to common problems encountered during chronic total occlusion angioplasty: the algorithms within the algorithm. Catheter Cardiovasc Interv 2019;93(2):286–97.
4. Alaswad K. Toolbox and inventory requirements for chronic total occlusion percutaneous coronary interventions. Interv Cardiol Clin 2012;1(3):281–97.
5. Brilakis ES, Mashayekhi K, Tsuchikane E, et al. Guiding principles for chronic total occlusion percutaneous coronary intervention. Circulation 2019;140(5):420–33.
6. Topol E. Textbook of interventional Cardiology. Eigth. Elsevier, Inc.; 2019.
7. Karacsonyi J, Tajti P, Rangan BV, et al. Randomized comparison of a Crossboss first versus standard wire escalation strategy for crossing coronary chronic total occlusions the crossboss first trial. JACC Cardiovasc Interv 2018;11(3):225–33.
8. Whitlow PL, Burke MN, Lombardi WL, et al. Use of a novel crossing and re-entry system in coronary chronic total occlusions that have failed standard crossing techniques results of the FAST-CTOs (facilitated antegrade steering technique in chronic total occlusions) trial. JACC Cardiovasc Interv 2012; 5(4):393–401.
9. Zhang J, Gao X, Kan J, et al. Intravascular ultrasound-guided versus angiography-guided implantation of drug-eluting stent in all-comers: the ULTIMATE trial. J Am Coll Cardiol 2018;72(24): 3126–37.
10. Tian N-L, Gami S-K, Ye F, et al. Angiographic and clinical comparisons of intravascular ultrasound-versus angiography-guided drug-eluting stent implantation for patients with chronic total occlusion lesions: two-year results from a randomised AIR-CTO study. Eurointervention 2015;10(12): 1409–17.

Antegrade Wire Escalation Case Selection and Strategies: Four Wires for Success

Anbukarasi Maran, MD*, Katrina A.E.L. Bidwell, MD

KEYWORDS

- Chronic total occlusion • Antegrade wire escalation • Percutaneous coronary intervention

---

KEY POINTS

- Patients appropriate for primary antegrade wire escalation (AWE) for CTO PCI are those with clear proximal cap, good-quality distal vessel, and short lesion length (<20 mm). Selected cases of CTO with long, straight segments or occlusive in-stent restenosis may also be appropriate for AWE.
- There are four basic families of wires to consider when using AWE: tapered tip, nontapered hydrophilic tip, penetrative tip, and highly penetrative tip wires. Within each family, there are numerous options available from various manufacturers.
- Especially for new operators, we recommend familiarizing oneself with one wire within each family; operators should only need four to five wires for AWE.
- An algorithmic approach to AWE includes stepwise escalation/de-escalation as needed; if unsuccessful, consideration of other strategies as part of the hybrid algorithm should be used.

 Video content accompanies this article at http://www.interventional.theclinics.com.

INTRODUCTION AND BACKGROUND

The North American Hybrid Algorithm (NAHA) has become the standard method for percutaneous intervention for coronary chronic total occlusions (CTO).[1] Once a patient has been identified as an appropriate candidate for intervention on a coronary CTO, the next step is to consider strategies for crossing the occlusion to perform percutaneous coronary intervention (PCI) according to the hybrid algorithm (Fig. 1). There are four general approaches available to operators for crossing CTOs: (1) antegrade wire escalation (AWE), (2) antegrade dissection and reentry, (3) retrograde wire escalation, and (4) retrograde wire escalation. AWE is usually the first step in the hybrid algorithm and involves crossing the proximal cap while within the true vessel lumen at all times. AWE is the most commonly used strategy[2,3] and is the most technically straightforward approach to crossing CTO vessels. Because of its technical simplicity it tends to be favored heavily by low- and intermediate-volume operators; it is also an indispensable skill set to even the most experienced of operators.

When evaluating a patient for primary AWE, the following angiographic characteristics should be considered:

- Proximal cap location and morphology
- Lesion length
- Quality of the distal vessel
- Distal landing zone

A clearly defined proximal cap favors a primary antegrade approach; the presence of tapered, unambiguous proximal cap often suggests the presence of a microchannel within the CTO segment. In contrast, a primary

---

Medical University of South Carolina, 30 Courtenay Drive, BM 326, MSC592, Charleston, SC 29425, USA
* Corresponding author.
E-mail address: maran@musc.edu

Intervent Cardiol Clin 10 (2021) 33–39
https://doi.org/10.1016/j.iccl.2020.09.008
2211-7458/21/Published by Elsevier Inc.

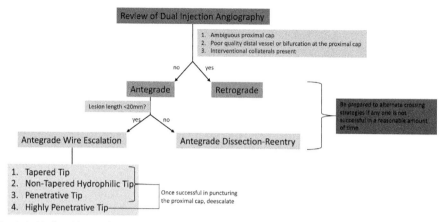

Fig. 1. The hybrid algorithm with antegrade wire escalation wire families.

retrograde approach tends to be more effective in the presence of a poorly defined, or ambiguous, cap. Shorter lesions, defined as those less than 20 mm, are more amenable to primary AWE with higher rates of successful wiring. Longer lesions, especially with associated calcium or tortuosity, often prove more difficult to cross and are associated with increased likelihood of subintimal guidewire entry; in such lesions a primary dissection/reentry strategy may prove more effective. Straight segments that are greater than 20 mm or those in which there is a suspected though-and-through microchannel may still be amenable to primary AWE.[4] The quality of the distal vessel or "landing zone" must also be evaluated. Small and diffusely diseased target vessels or those with bifurcations distal to the cap are less ideal for AWE, and the presence of good-quality collateral vessels that are considered crossable by the operator should prompt consideration of a primary retrograde approach when antegrade strategies are unfavorable because of distal or proximal cap ambiguity. AWE is usually the primary strategy in cases of occlusive in-stent restenosis given the defined vessel course. Finally, the operator must be prepared to rapidly transition to a dissection and reentry strategy in all cases of attempted AWE given the likelihood of tracking in the subintimal space requiring an alternative strategy to simply wiring the true lumen for reproducible success.

In addition to the NAHA, there are several other algorithms available to aid operators in crossing strategy selection. The Japan-CTO score has become widely used; it considers similar angiographic characteristics to the NAHA in addition to whether or not treatment of the vessel segment in question had been attempted previously (Table 1).[5] Lesions are stratified as easy, intermediate, difficult, or very difficult to cross based on numerical score. AWE is most successful with anatomy with a J-CTO score of 0 or 1; in the original literature, around 40% of lesions fell into this category.[5,6]

The key principle of the NAHA is that "anatomy dictates strategy," and one should be willing and skilled to switch strategies when one is not working.[1] In general, lesions should be able to be crossed with the appropriate strategy within 30 minutes.[5] Failing to achieve progress in a reasonable amount of time should prompt the operator to consider alternating strategies, whether that be by exchanging wires or changing crossing method.

DISCUSSION
The Different Families of Wires
The current armamentarium of interventional wires on the market can prove daunting, with respect to the number of options and upfront equipment cost. With respect to AWE specifically, we consider four groups or families of wires to be essential. There are multiple proprietary options available from different manufacturers in each category; however, by focusing on families of wires for a specific purpose as opposed to particular models, an operator should be able to pare their toolbox down to four or five wires only for AWE. The following are the general classes of wires useful for AWE (Table 2):

1. Tapered tip: This is the first wire used in straightforward lesions when workhorse wire with microcatheter is unsuccessful or unlikely to cross; these are particularly useful for traversing microchannels, which may not be visible. These are nondrilling wires that do

Table 1
The Japan CTO score template

Variable	Point Value
Previously failed lesion	No (0)
	Yes (1)
Stump type: any dimple or tapering indicating the direction of the true lumen is considered tapered	Tapered (0)
	Blunt (1)
Calcification: regardless of severity, any calcium present in the CTO segment	Absent (0)
	Present (1)
Bending: one point is assigned if there is any bending >45° within the CTO segment	Absent (0)
	Present (1)
Occlusion length	<20 mm (0)
	≥20 mm (1)
Difficulty score based on point total	
	Easy: 0
	Intermediate: 1
	Difficult: 2
	Very difficult: ≥3

not have much body and knuckle when faced with resistance (ie, are considered "softer" guidewires). Examples include Fielder XT (Asahi Intecc, Seto-Shi, Japan), Fielder XT-A (Asahi Intecc), and Fighter (Boston Scientific, Marlborough, MA). Many operators forgo this step and move directly to the next class, because data suggest wire crossing is more successful in the next group in CTO PCI.

2. Nontapered hydrophilic tip: Wires in this grouping have a hydrophilic coating (or jacket) throughout the wire except for the distal microcone-shaped, noncoated tip. This allows higher penetration efficacy, despite being more flexible. Similar to group 1, these are nondrilling wires for locating and traversing nonvisible microchannels and are considered to be "stiff, jacketed" guidewires. Examples

Table 2
The four families of wires for AWE

Wire Group	Representative Wires (Classic Example in Bold)	Notes
Tapered tip	*Fielder XT* (Asahi Intecc), Fielder XT-A (Asahi Intecc), Fighter (Boston Scientific), Banditä (Teleflex)	Generally used first to track a microchannel
Nontapered hydrophilic tip	*Pilot 200* (Abbott Vascular), Choice PT Graphix (Boston Scientific), Raider (Teleflex), Gladius Mongo[a] (Asahi Intecc)	Preferred if course of vessel is not known
Penetrative tip	Gaia (Asahi Intecc), Gaia 2 (Asahi Intecc), Gaia 3 (Asahi Intecc), Judo 6 (Boston Scientific)	Preferred if the course of the vessel is short or well understood
Highly penetrative tip	*Confianza Pro 12* (Asahi Intecc), Hornet 14 (Boston Scientific), Miraclebros 12 (Asahi Intecc), Astato XS 20 (Asahi Intecc)	Scratch-and-go

[a] Can also be used as a knuckle wire.

include Pilot 200 (Abbott Vascular, St. Paul, MN), Gladius and Gladius Mongo (Asahi Intecc), and Raider (Teleflex, Wayne, PA).

3. Penetrative tip: If attempting to locate a microchannel is unsuccessful, wires with a more penetrative tip provide increased force to puncture a cap impenetrable with the previously mentioned wires in particularly resistant and calcified lesions. These wires are designed to provide some tactile feedback when the wire exits the lumen, although this may be difficult to discern early in an operator's experience. Great care is required to ensure the wire remains in the vessel architecture before following with the next step in gear. This is necessary with the "scratch and go" technique, wherein the operator escalates the wires from groups 1 to 3 and "scratches" the proximal cap to engage the lesion or the vessel's subintimal plane just proximal to the cap, which may require highly penetrative wires. These wires should not be used to traverse lesions given, as their name suggests, their highly penetrative nature and likelihood of causing perforation. As such, this is followed by rapid deescalation to a wire in one of the other groups once successful in puncturing the proximal cap to ensure a wire with less penetration power tracks within the vessel architecture. Examples include Confianza Pro 12 (Asahi Intecc), Hornet 14 (Boston Scientific), and Astato 20 (Asahi Intecc).

The wires are listed in the order that they should be used and represent escalation in terms of tip load and therefore penetrative force. Among patients with a J-CTO score of 0 to 1, escalation past soft guidewires should be expected about 50% of the time, with successful AWE in around 75% of these cases with the use of the full set of guidewires.[2] If the wire still cannot cross the proximal cap, intravascular ultrasound (IVUS) is useful to further characterize the anatomy of the CTO and identify any microchannels.

APPLICATION

Effective wiring technique is the key to success for CTO PCI in general. The following techniques are useful in AWE.

Drilling involves controlled rotation of the guidewire in either direction to advance. Small, less than 90° rotations and a small tip bend are important so as not to create a large subintimal

space.[4] Intermediate stiffness wires (3–6 g) are used initially, such as the Pilot 200 (Abbott Vascular) or the Gaia family (Asahi Intecc). Nonpolymer-jacketed wires (eg, the Gaia family) are intended to provide additional tactile feedback. When needed, the operator uses gradual step-up of the wire stiffness according to the lesion complexity, being mindful that tip load and degree of tactile feedback are inversely related, particularly with polymer-jacketed wires.

Loose tissue tracking is intended to traverse loose tissue segments in the proximal cap and is conceptually similar to how one would cross a lesion in an acute myocardial infarction case. The operator shapes the distal 1 to 2 mm of a nontapered intermediate-strength wire into a 45° to 60° bend so that the wire tip is controlled and directed in such a way that it advances though tissue planes but does not penetrate hard atherosclerotic plaque.[7] If the intermediate-strength wire is not successful in crossing the space between fibrous tissues, escalation to a wire with a stiffer tapered tip end is considered. When loose tissue tracking fails, the wire is manipulated into the intimal plaque or subintimal space.

Adequate guide support is of nearly equal importance to wire selection in ensuring the success of AWE and cannot be overemphasized. This is accomplished with a microcatheter or a guide catheter extension as appropriate. A microcatheter should be used in AWE attempts to provide wire support and increase tip stiffness and allowing the operator to reshape the wire as needed and facilitating guidewire exchange without losing wire position, and to protect the proximal vessel from injury because of multiple guidewire exchanges with the properties described herein.

CASE STUDIES
Case 1
The patient is a 68-year-old man with hypertension, diabetes, and coronary artery disease status post multiple prior PCIs. He presented to his general cardiologist with typical exertional angina such that it interfered with his activities of daily living despite optimal medical therapy. His medications included isosorbide mononitrate, 60 mg daily; ranolazine, 1000 mg twice daily; metoprolol succinate, 25 mg daily; lisinopril, 40 mg daily; and aspirin, 81 mg daily. He was then taken for coronary angiography and was found to have a CTO of the left anterior descending artery (LAD). He did not have any significant right to left collaterals. He was

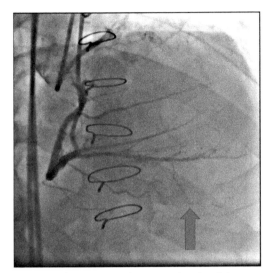

Fig. 2. Dual angiogram demonstrating the right coronary artery with right ventricular marginal branch (*blue arrow*).

subsequently referred to our institution for consideration of CTO PCI.

- JCTO score: blunt cap, greater than 20 mm = 2 points (difficult).
- Access: right femoral artery, left femoral artery. Antegrade guide: extra backup, 3.75. Retrograde guide: hockey stick.
- Dual angiogram (**Figs. 2** and **3**, Video 1): LAD proximal CTO within previously placed stent, right coronary artery (RCA)

with mild in-stent restenosis. There is a marginal branch providing epicardial collaterals to the distal LAD.

AWE with a Corsair microcatheter (Asahi Intecc) and Fielder guidewire (Asahi Intecc) was done; the wire went to the level of the stent and was not able to be advanced (Video 2). Next, a Judo 3 wire (Boston Scientific) was used to cross the distal cap (scratch and go, Video 3) and wire deescalation to the Fielder was done with successful advancement to the distal vessel (Video 4). Position was confirmed with IVUS, which also demonstrated severe diffuse fibrofatty plaque. The areas distal and proximal to the previous stent were treated with drug-eluting stents. The stents were postdilated with a 4.0 × 20 noncompliant balloon. Final angiogram demonstrated excellent stent expansion without dissection and TIMI III flow, which was confirmed with IVUS (**Fig. 4**).

Case 2

The patient is a 47-year-old man with a history of type II diabetes and premature coronary artery disease status post coronary artery bypass grafting with saphenous vein graft to the RCA known to be occluded, saphenous vein graft to the obtuse marginal, and left internal mammary graft to the LAD with subsequent PCI. He presented for evaluation of chronic stable angina despite optimal medical therapy. His medications included isosorbide mononitrate, 30 mg daily; losartan, 50 mg daily; metoprolol succinate, 100 mg daily; ranolazine, 1000 mg twice daily; rosuvastatin, 40 mg; aspirin, 81 mg daily;

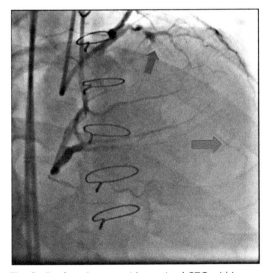

Fig. 3. Dual angiogram with proximal CTO within previously placed stent in the LAD (*red arrow*). There is a marginal branch providing epicardial collaterals to the distal LAD (*blue arrow*).

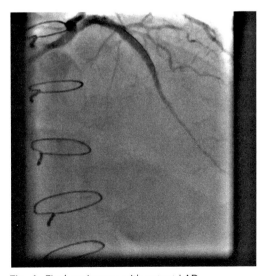

Fig. 4. Final angiogram with patent LAD.

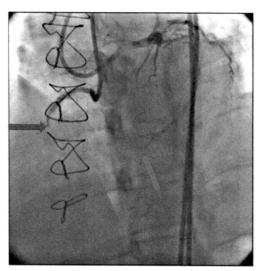

Fig. 5. LAD, left circumflex, RCA all with mid-vessel CTO. Within the RCA, the proximal cap (*red arrow*) and distal cap (*blue arrow*) are seen with the vessel reconstituting distally.

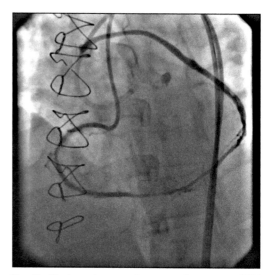

Fig. 7. Final angiogram demonstrating patent RCA back filling a jump graft to the obtuse marginal.

- Dual angiogram (Fig. 5): LAD, left circumflex, RCA all with mid-vessel CTO.

The Amplatz Left guide was reinforced with an 8F catheter Trapliner and a runthrough wire was placed in the mid-RCA. Next, with a Corsair 135 cm microcatheter (Asahi Intecc), a Fielder XT guidewire (Asahi Intecc) was used to probe the proximal cap but was unsuccessful in crossing. Next, a Pilot 200 (Abbott Vascular) was used but was unsuccessful in crossing. A Gladius Mongo (Asahi Intecc) wire was used and knuckled behind the previously placed stent struts and crossed into the distal posterior descending branch. The Corsair was exchanged for a CrossBoss over-the-wire catheter (Boston Scientific); however, the CrossBoss could not get back intraluminally (Fig. 6, Video 5). Using a Twin-Pass Torque catheter (Teleflex) a Gladius Mongo knuckle was initiated in the mid-vessel, proximal to the stent, and was passed within the stent struts into the posterior descending branch (Video 6). This was confirmed with IVUS, which showed severe neointimal hyperplasia throughout the distal and mid-vessel stent. The distal RCA was treated with plain old balloon angioplasty with 2 × 40 and the stented segments were treated with laser atherectomy with a 0.9 catheter at 60/60 rate and fluency. Next, balloon angioplasty of the stented segments was done with 2.5 and 3.5 noncompliant balloons. The final angiogram demonstrated TIMI III flow in the RCA and its branches, back filling a jump graft to the obtuse marginal (Fig. 7, Video 7).

clopidogrel, 75 mg daily; and chlorthalidone 25 mg daily.

- JCTO score: length greater than 20 mm, blunt cap, calcification = 3 (very difficult).
- Access: right femoral artery, left femoral artery. Antegrade guide: Amplatz Left, 0.75. Retrograde guide: extra backup, 3.5.

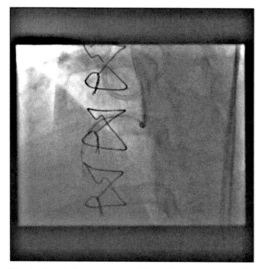

Fig. 6. Escalating support with guide extension in the RCA with a blunt-tip dissection tool and a knuckle wire.

SUMMARY

AWE is the crossing technique of choice for short, focal, noncalcified straight segments of CTO lesions. Although many options in terms of equipment are available to operators and can become quickly overwhelming, the focus on four general wire types helps to simplify the selection process. Operators should not need more than four to five wires for AWE. Attempt crossing with these select wires and if not successful, quickly move on to the next strategy.

CLINICS CARE POINTS

- Patients appropriate for primary AWE for CTO PCI are those with clear proximal cap, good-quality distal vessel, and short lesion length (<20 mm). Selected cases of CTO with long, straight segments or occlusive in-stent restenosis may also be appropriate for AWE.
- There are four basic families of wires to consider when using AWE: tapered tip, nontapered hydrophilic tip, penetrative tip, and highly penetrative tip wires. Within each family, there are numerous options available from various manufacturers.
- It is important to develop familiarity with one wire within each family to avoid overwhelming oneself and the cardiac catheterization laboratory budget by purchasing wires of similar function from different manufacturers.
- An algorithmic approach to AWE includes stepwise escalation/de-escalation as needed; if unsuccessful, consideration of other strategies as part of the hybrid algorithm should be used.

DISCLOSURE

The authors have nothing to disclose.

SUPPLEMENTARY DATA

Supplementary data related to this article can be found online at https://doi.org/10.1016/j.iccl.2020.09.008.

REFERENCES

1. Brilakis ES, Grantham JA, Rinfret S, et al. A percutaneous treatment algorithm for crossing coronary chronic total occlusions. JACC Cardiovasc Interv 2012. https://doi.org/10.1016/j.jcin.2012.02.006.
2. Maeremans J, Knaapen P, Stuijfzand WJ, et al. Antegrade wire escalation for chronic total occlusions in coronary arteries: simple algorithms as a key to success. J Cardiovasc Med 2016. https://doi.org/10.2459/JCM.0000000000000340.
3. Karatasakis A, Tarar MNJ, Karmpaliotis D, et al. Guidewire and microcatheter utilization patterns during antegrade wire escalation in chronic total occlusion percutaneous coronary intervention: insights from a contemporary multicenter registry. Catheter Cardiovasc Interv 2017. https://doi.org/10.1002/ccd.26568.
4. Brilakis ES. 4 - Antegrade Wire Escalation: The Foundation of CTO PCI. In: Brilakis ES, editor. Manual of Coronary Chronic Total Occlusion Interventions. St Louis (MO): Academic Press; 2014. p. 95-120.
5. Morino Y, Abe M, Morimoto T, et al. Predicting successful guidewire crossing through chronic total occlusion of native coronary lesions within 30 minutes. JACC Cardiovasc Interv 2011. https://doi.org/10.1016/j.jcin.2010.09.024.
6. Brilakis ES, Banerjee S, Karmpaliotis D, et al. Procedural outcomes of chronic total occlusion percutaneous coronary intervention: a report from the NCDR (National Cardiovascular Data Registry). JACC Cardiovasc Interv 2015. https://doi.org/10.1016/j.jcin.2014.08.014.
7. Dash D. Guidewire crossing techniques in coronary chronic total occlusion intervention: A to Z. Indian Heart J 2016. https://doi.org/10.1016/j.ihj.2016.02.019.

Antegrade Dissection and Reentry: Tools and Techniques

R. Michael Wyman, MD

KEYWORDS

- Chronic total occlusions • Percutaneous coronary intervention • Antegrade approach
- Dissection/reentry • BridgePoint device

KEY POINTS

- Antegrade dissection and reentry is an essential component of chronic total occlusion percutaneous coronary intervention.
- Previous techniques (STAR and its modifications) have been limited by low success rates and a lack of control over the site of reentry.
- The BridgePoint device was developed specifically for antegrade dissection and reentry and allows for efficient subintimal tracking and targeted reentry.
- Evolution of technique in conjunction with use of the BridgePoint device has resulted in an expansion of the anatomic subsets for which antegrade dissection and reentry can be successfully used.

INTRODUCTION

Coronary artery chronic total occlusions (CTO) remain the most challenging lesion subset for percutaneous intervention. Despite a growing body of evidence relating to poor long-term outcomes in patients with CTOs[1,2] and favorable effects of revascularization,[3,4] attempt rates in the United States remain low.[5] Reasons for this include historical perceptions related to low success rates and prolonged procedure times, and operator anxiety about working in the coronary subintimal space.

Multiple advances in technique and technology, many of them originally developed by Japanese operators, have led to significant improvements in procedural success.[6] Guidewire and microcatheter advances, and technique iterations, have refined the strategies of antegrade wire escalation, retrograde wiring, and retrograde dissection reentry to allow reproducible outcomes in the hands of highly skilled operators.[7] However, this experience has not lent itself to widespread adoption internationally for

three reasons: (1) the lack of a simplified and teachable strategy for how to approach any given anatomic situation; (2) the lack of emphasis on time (and radiation) efficiency; and (3) no previously available option for consistently successful antegrade dissection and reentry.

The hybrid approach to CTO percutaneous coronary intervention (PCI) was developed in response to these unmet needs.[8] An algorithm based on anatomic lesion characteristics defines the primary and subsequent secondary (tertiary and so forth) strategies (**Fig. 1**). The approach requires familiarity with all four potential options for wire crossing (**Fig. 2**), and just as importantly a willingness to move quickly and seamlessly from one strategy to another if failure modes are encountered. Antegrade dissection and reentry is as integral a component of wire crossing in the hybrid approach as any of the other three (antegrade wiring, retrograde wiring, retrograde dissection and reentry), yet it has suffered from inadequate tools to consistently achieve high levels of success. The lack

This article originally appeared in *Interventional Cardiology Clinics*, Volume 1, Issue 3, July 2012.
Cardiovascular Interventional Research, Torrance Memorial Medical Center, 3445 Pacific Coast Highway, Suite 100, Torrance, CA 90505, USA
E-mail address: rmwcor@gmail.com

Intervent Cardiol Clin 10 (2021) 41–50
https://doi.org/10.1016/j.iccl.2020.10.001

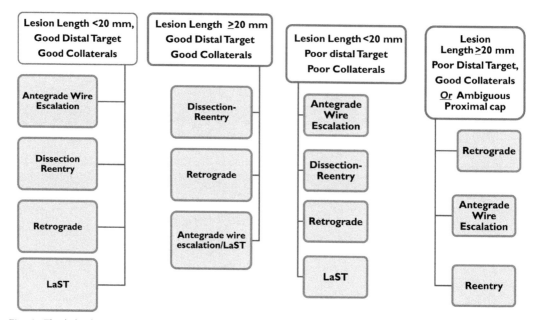

Fig. 1. The hybrid approach algorithm. Initial and subsequent strategies based on anatomic characteristics.

of wire and catheter control over both ends of the CTO segment (as is available in retrograde dissection and reentry) has traditionally made successful reentry from the antegrade direction a challenge. The BridgePoint device (Bridge-Point Medical, Plymouth, MN, USA), which is the only coronary CTO product to have been developed specifically for gaining reentry into the true lumen from the subintimal space, has now allowed antegrade dissection and reentry

to take it's appropriate place as an essential crossing option in the hybrid approach to CTO PCI.

ANATOMY

An important precept of the hybrid approach is that anatomic characteristics of the CTO dictate initial and subsequent strategy (see Fig. 1). A typical anatomic substrate that would lend itself

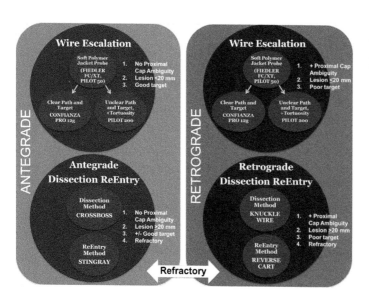

Fig. 2. The four crossing options for CTO intervention. Associated favorable anatomic indicators are listed to the right.

to antegrade dissection and reentry as a primary strategy includes the following (Fig. 3):

- A well defined proximal cap
- Lesion length greater than 20 mm
- Moderate caliber distal vessel
- No large branches at the distal cap.

Other traditional indicators of CTO success, such as the presence of bridging collaterals, very long lesion length, tortuosity, and calcification, have little or no impact on the decision algorithm. In addition, as discussed later, a rapid evolution in technique has allowed for a significant expansion of the anatomic inclusion criteria for antegrade dissection reentry, such that an ambiguous proximal cap and diffusely diseased distal vessel become appropriate lesion subsets for primary attempts.

PREPROCEDURE PLANNING

As with any CTO intervention, meticulous preparation is a key to success. This includes physician, catheter laboratory, and patient-specific planning. The physician needs to be comfortable with the commonly used CTO skillsets (not limited to antegrade dissection and reentry), which include

- Advanced guide support techniques
- Specialized microcatheter (Tornus and Corsair; Asahi Intecc, Nagoya, Japan) manipulations

- Wire knuckling
- Wire puncturing techniques
- Balloon anchoring and trapping
- Contrast and radiation management.

The catheter laboratory should be well prepared in terms of equipment availability (preferably with the most frequently used CTO-specific gear on a separate "CTO cart") and a supportive and actively engaged staff.

Patient preparation includes detailed study of the diagnostic angiogram before proceeding, which obviates performing procedures in an ad hoc fashion. Careful attention should be paid to all of the aforementioned anatomic features and vessel take-off from the aorta, proximal tortuosity and disease, branches for anchoring, previously placed stents, donor vessel characteristics, collateral access, and so forth. Optimal imaging during the procedure is essential, which primarily necessitates the use of contralateral injections to visualize the distal vessel. Even in circumstances where ipsilateral collaterals are dominant and only faint contralateral collaterals are apparent, it is strongly recommended that dual access be obtained to prepare for the likely eventuality of loss of forward collateral visualization. This is particularly true for antegrade dissection and reentry, wherein antegrade contrast injections are strictly avoided to minimize enlargement of the subintimal space. Use of available state-of-the-art imaging equipment is also advisable, in terms of image quality and minimization of radiation dose.

PROCEDURAL APPROACH

Antegrade dissection reentry was originally described, in the coronary tree, as the subintimal tracking and reentry (STAR) technique.[9] As in peripheral (primarily superficial femoral artery [SFA]) CTO procedures, a knuckled wire is passed through and beyond the CTO segment, with distal true lumen access dependent on unpredictable and uncontrolled reentry, often into a small distal branch. Reconstruction of larger, more proximal branches, to preserve myocardial perfusion and enable adequate outflow (and thus proximal patency) can then be performed by "refenestration" techniques with polymer jacketed wires. Although an adequate angiographic result can be achieved, questions about true myocardial perfusion and long-term patency persist, and the authors themselves consider this to be a true bail-out, last chance technique, advising in addition against its use in the left anterior descending,

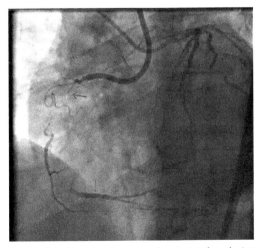

Fig. 3. A right coronary artery chronic total occlusion with favorable anatomic characteristics for primary antegrade dissection and reentry. The proximal cap (*thick arrow*) is well defined. The lesion length is greater than 20 mm. The distal vessel (*thin arrow*) reentry zone has an adequate caliber and there is no significant branch nearby.

where multiple sidebranches (ie, septal perforators) could be sheared off and not recovered.

Additional iterations of the STAR technique have been described, including contrast enhanced and mini-STAR,[10] yet these remain saddled with suboptimal control over the reentry site location, and relatively low rates of reentry success.

Despite these challenges, it has been clear for many years that any successful approach to CTO intervention requires the use of the subintimal space in a significant number of cases. The CTO experience in peripheral vessels, the Japanese operators' development of subintimal techniques for retrograde dissection and reentry (CART and reverse CART), and the failure of previous CTO niche devices that focused on true lumen crossing (eg, frontrunner, SafeCross) have all strongly reinforced this concept.

The BridgePoint device was specifically developed to take advantage of this frequent need for subintimal tracking to gain successful distal lumen access. There are three components to the system:

1. The CrossBoss catheter (Fig. 4): a multiple wire coiled shaft with a 0.014-in compatible through lumen, ending distally in a blunt, polished 1-mm distal tip. A proximal rotating device is rapidly spun outside the body by the operator, with gentle forward catheter pressure.

2. The Stingray balloon catheter (Fig. 5): an over-the-wire, 2.5-mm wide, flat balloon catheter that self-orients within the subintimal space. Two 180-degree opposed ports then allow controlled wire exit toward either the luminal space or the adventitial surface. Each port is located just proximal to a radiopaque marker.

3. The Stingray guidewire (see Fig. 5): a 12-g force wire with a shallow preformed angulated distal tip, and a 1-mm extruded segment that acts to catch tissue and penetrate through the subintima and into the true lumen.

A typical antegrade dissection reentry procedure with the BridgePoint device (Fig. 6) involves advancement of the CrossBoss catheter over a workhorse wire to the proximal cap, retraction of the wire into the catheter lumen, then rapid rotation of the catheter through the body of the CTO. The CrossBoss tracks into a distal true luminal position in 20% to 30% of cases,[11] but when the more frequent subintimal position is achieved, beyond the distal cap at an appropriate reentry position the guidewire is advanced and the catheter exchanged out for the Stingray balloon. This is brought into position over the guidewire and inflated to 3 to 4 atm. Visualization of the flat balloon is extremely important to enable orientation in relation to the distal vessel lumen, and to

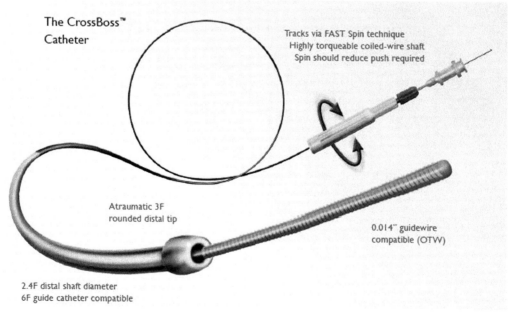

The CrossBoss™ Catheter

Tracks via FAST Spin technique
Highly torqueable coiled-wire shaft
Spin should reduce push required

Atraumatic 3F rounded distal tip

0.014" guidewire compatible (OTW)

2.4F distal shaft diameter
6F guide catheter compatible

Fig. 4. The CrossBoss catheter. (Image provided courtesy of Boston Scientific. ©2020 Boston Scientific Corporation or its affiliates. All rights reserved.)

The Stingray™ Catheter
& The Stingray™ Guidewire

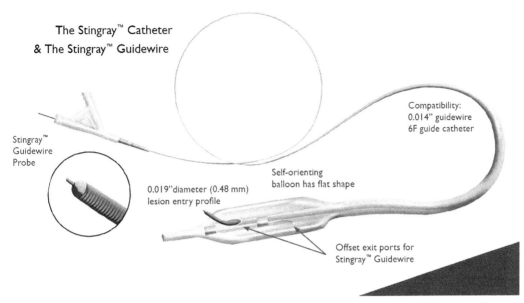

Stingray™
Guidewire
Probe

0.019"diameter (0.48 mm)
lesion entry profile

Self-orienting
balloon has flat shape

Compatibility:
0.014" guidewire
6F guide catheter

Offset exit ports for
Stingray™ Guidewire

Fig. 5. The Stingray balloon catheter and the Stingray wire. (Image provided courtesy of Boston Scientific. ©2020 Boston Scientific Corporation or its affiliates. All rights reserved.)

determine the optimal view for reentry. This necessitates a meticulous preparation with 100% contrast. A contralateral angiogram is performed to demonstrate the balloon–vessel relationship, and the Stingray guidewire is then advanced and exited through the appropriate (luminal) port, with a direct puncture technique. A contralateral injection is again used to confirm the position of the wire in the lumen; the wire is rotated 180 degrees (away from the opposite wall) and advanced distally into the vessel. The Stingray balloon is then removed and an over-the-wire balloon or microcatheter is advanced, with subsequent exchange of the Stingray wire for a workhorse wire, over which all routine ballooning and stenting can then be performed.

Although the described technique is successful in many cases, extensive experience with the device by high-volume operators, and their collaboration on technique iteration, has led to multiple advances that have markedly influenced the anatomic opportunities for which the device is useful. These situations can be broadly grouped into overcoming difficulty with advancement of gear to the "base of operations" (ie, just beyond the distal cap for antegrade procedures) and overcoming challenges with reentry.

Gear Hangup
The proximal cap and body of the CTO are sometimes resistant to passage of the Cross-Boss. In addition, an ambiguous or flush occluded proximal cap does not allow for entry

of the CrossBoss into the CTO body. Finally, the CrossBoss can track into a side branch within the CTO segment, before arriving at the distal cap. These challenges can all be dealt with using similar techniques. For an ambiguous or resistant proximal cap, a stiff penetrating wire (either tapered tip hydrophilic or nontapered jacketed) is used to make initial progress over a very short distance (no more than 5–10 mm) using either the CrossBoss or another microcatheter as support. Longer traverses with the stiff wire, especially if followed by the support catheter, should be assiduously avoided because the potential for vessel perforation is enhanced. Instead, a knuckled wire (described in more detail later) is used to traverse most of the CTO segment, although not beyond the distal cap to the reentry site. The CrossBoss catheter is used to make the final subintimal dissection distally. This allows for a more refined dissection (with less enlargement of the space) while providing an adequate pathway for subsequent advancement of the Stingray catheter.

Reentry Challenges
These are represented by either loss of distal visualization of the reentry segment, usually by a compressive subintimal hematoma, or by a small diffusely diseased vessel beyond the distal cap. In the first case, preventive measures are a key: avoiding creation of a large subintimal space with antegrade injections, aggressive wire manipulation, or extended knuckling, and

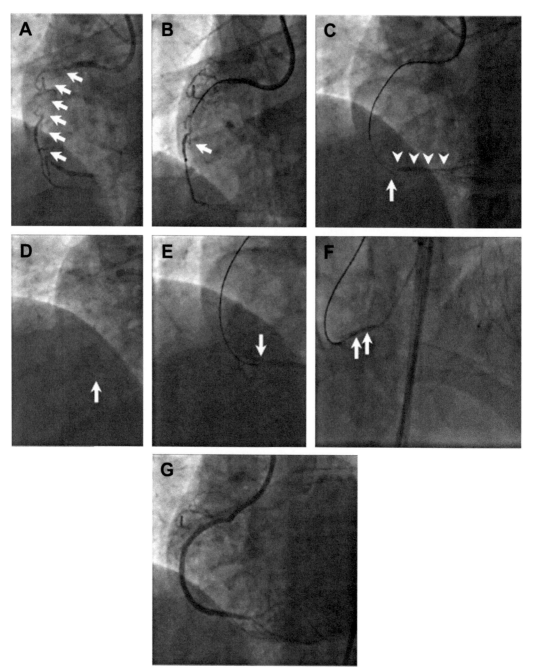

Fig. 6. Antegrade dissection reentry in a right coronary artery CTO (*A*, *arrows* denoting length of occlusion segment) using the BridgePoint device. The CrossBoss catheter is spun rapidly through the CTO (*B*, *C* with *arrow* at tip of crossboss and *arrowheads* at planned re-entry site) to a subintimal position just beyond the distal cap. The Stingray balloon (*D* with two radiopaque markers at *arrow*) is exchanged for and reentry is accomplished with the Stingray wire (*E*, *F*, with *arrows* showing wire puncture and reentry). After predilation and stenting, the vessel is recanalized (*G*). (*From* Whitlow PL, Burke MN, Lombardi WL, et al. Use of a novel crossing and re-entry system in coronary chronic total occlusions that have failed standard crossing techniques: results of the FAST-CTOs trial. JACC Cardiovasc Interv 2012;5:393–401.)

instead using the Crossboss catheter as detailed previously. If a hematoma forms, aspiration of the subintimal space with a separate over-the-wire system can be attempted, although currently available over-the-wire balloons in the United States do not allow for simultaneous positioning with the Stingray in an 8Fr catheter guide.

In the case of a small and diffusely diseased distal vessel, a wire swap technique is very useful (Fig. 7): after initial puncturing into the lumen with the Stingray wire (which is not designed for finessed advancement through diseased vessels), the wire is removed and, with the Stingray balloon still inflated, swapped out for a jacketed wire. The latter is then directed out the same exit port, allowing access into the lumen and manipulation into the distal vessel with enhanced success.

The Art of the Knuckle

A knuckled or looped wire has been used for many years in peripheral CTO intervention for rapid advancement through the subintimal space. This technique has now become an essential component of subintimal tracking in coronary CTO PCI for antegrade and retrograde approaches. A knuckled wire has the advantage of quickly and safely traversing occlusive

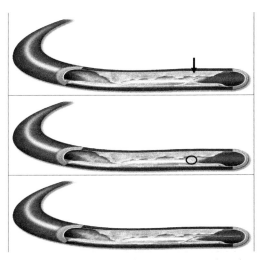

Fig. 7. The wire swap technique. An initial stick is made with the Stingray wire through the distal port of the Stingray catheter (*top*), from the subintimal space and into the lumen. The disease beyond the distal cap limits further advancement of the wire and it is removed (*middle*) with the balloon position maintained. A polymer jacketed wire is advanced and accesses the same exit port (*bottom*) with easier manipulation into the distal vessel. (Image provided courtesy of Boston Scientific. ©2020 Boston Scientific Corporation or its affiliates. All rights reserved.)

anatomy, particularly in those situations where the course of the vessel is not well understood. In comparison, use of stiff, tapered tip wires to cover the same geography can be time consuming and prone to perforation. This is because the adventitia, although very distensible in response to blunt force delivered over a large surface area (ie, the knuckle wire), can be punctured easily with a penetrating force delivered at a single focus (ie, a stiff tapered tip wire).

The most frequently used wires for knuckling in the coronary tree are polymer jacketed wires, either soft (with or without a tapered tip) or stiff and nontapered. The goal is to catch the tip of the wire (whether or not it has been preshaped into the classic "umbrella handle") on tissue within the vessel architecture, so that a loop is formed in a more proximal segment of the wire as it is advanced. This working aspect of the knuckle is often at the junction between the radiopaque coils and the stiffer more radiolucent part of the wire (Fig. 8). At times, depending on vessel tortuosity and calcification, the amount of force necessary to advance the knuckle can be significant. This sensation runs counter to even the most experienced interventionalists' concept of wire advancement through the coronary tree. However, as long as the size of the loop is controlled, such that it is not significantly larger than the perceived diameter of the vessel, this forward force remains safe and time efficient. Loop size management depends on the type of wire used (soft jacketed wires tending to form smaller loops) and on the relationship between the support catheter and the knuckle. If the loop becomes too large, advancement of the support catheter and retraction of the wire (at times completely back into the catheter) with subsequent reknuckling often controls loop size.

Additional advantages of knuckling include its ability to bypass areas of resistance met by more focused catheters (as discussed previously in relation to CrossBoss techniques), and its tendency to avoid entry into sidebranches that are a smaller diameter than the main vessel.

Limited Antegrade Subintimal Tracking and Redirection

A more recently described antegrade dissection reentry technique,[12] limited antegrade subintimal tracking and redirection (LAST) involves the advancement of a knuckled wire down to, but not beyond (as in STAR), the distal cap. A support catheter is then brought to the same position and a stiff wire (either polymer jacketed, nontapered, or nonjacketed and tapered),

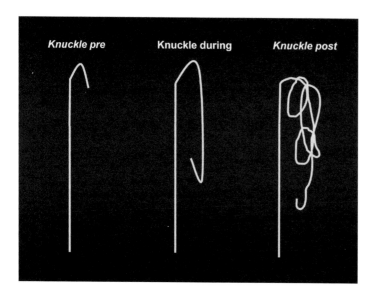

Fig. 8. The knuckle wire. Traditional "umbrella handle" shaping of wire before entry (*left*). The working loop of the knuckle (*middle*) is more proximal, often at the junction of the soft and stiffer segments. After removal, the wire is frequently quite deformed (*right*).

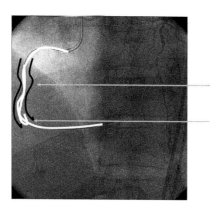

Fig. 9. Limited antegrade subintimal tracking.

Unsuccessful wiring of CTO

1. *Knuckle wire for limited distance to change wiring location/modify lesion*
2. *Redirect path with confianza pro 12g and/or pilot 200*

usually with a more exaggerated tip bend, is used to try and reenter the distal true lumen (**Fig. 9**). Theoretically, the wire should engage the tissue in the distal body of the CTO to gain luminal entry, rather than attempting a true reentry from the subintimal space beyond the distal cap. This technique, as noted by its acronym, is also a final bailout option should all other strategies fail, but one that has advantages over STAR and has met with fairly good anecdotal success.

Fig. 10 is a schematic depiction comparing the various antegrade dissection and reentry techniques. LAST has more potential control over the site of reentry than STAR, but neither has the predictable and accurate control of BridgePoint nor the same level of success.

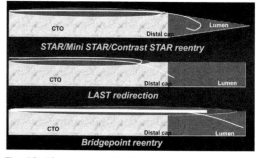

Fig. 10. Three antegrade dissection and reentry techniques. The BridgePoint device allows for the only true control over reentry.

Table 1
Technical success and MACE in the FAST-CTO trial compared with other CTO device trials

	FAST-CTOs	Crosser	SafeCross	Frontrunner
No. of patients	147	125	116	107
Technical success	77%	61%	54%	56%
30-d MACE	4.8%	8.8%	6.9%	8%

CLINICAL RESULTS

A number of published reports have delineated the worldwide experience with the BridgePoint device, from first-in-man descriptions[13] to European and isolated case reports.[14,15] The most comprehensive data come from the recently published outcomes of the US Facilitated Antegrade Steering Technique in Chronic Total Occlusions (FAST-CTO) trial.[11] A total of 150 refractory CTOs, defined as either a failed attempt within the last year or failed wiring attempts during the index procedure, were treated with the device. The primary end point was successful placement of a guidewire within the distal true lumen, with secondary end points of fluoroscopy and procedure time. The safety end point was major adverse cardiac event (MACE) out to 30 days. Anatomic exclusion criteria included saphenous vein graft, in-stent, or aorto-ostial lesions, and a small distal vessel caliber (<1.5 mm) or large branch at the distal cap. There was no exclusion for lesion length, which by Core lab QCA measurement was 22 mm, similar to most other CTO device and registry studies.

Technical success results compared with the historical control of previous CTO device trials are shown in Table 1. The success rate of 77% compared favorably and led to Food and Drug Administration approval. Equally important, there was a definite learning curve noted (Fig. 11), with success rates in the latter half of the trial population increasing to 86%. Insofar as many of the investigators had no prior experience with the device, familiarity clearly led to content.

Fluoroscopy and procedure time were 105 and 44 minutes, significantly less than the historical controls. Thirty-day MACE was 4.8%, with two late deaths (>16 days) unrelated to the procedure and five device-related perforations (3.4%), none of which required pericardiocentesis or surgery.

SUMMARY

Percutaneous intervention on CTOs in the coronary tree, although often clinically indicated, has been inhibited because of the perception of low success rates; long procedure times; high radiation exposure; and safety concerns, particularly in regards to operator comfort levels with working in the subintimal space. With the development of an objective and teachable strategy for approaching CTO intervention safely and efficiently (the hybrid approach), many of these concerns can be alleviated. Antegrade dissection and reentry is an essential component of the hybrid approach, largely because of the availability of the BridgePoint device. Initial experience with this device, and subsequent rapid evolution of technique, has led to a progressive expansion of the anatomic subsets for which the device can allow successful recanalization of these difficult lesions.

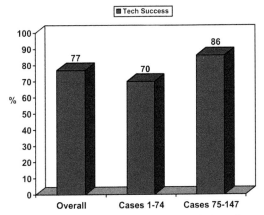

Fig. 11. The learning curve in the FAST-CTO trial.

REFERENCES

1. Hannan EL, Wu C, Walford G, et al. Incomplete revascularization in the era of drug eluting stents: impact on adverse outcomes. JACC Cardiovasc Interv 2009;2:17–25.
2. Claessen BE, van der Schaaf RJ, Verouden NJ, et al. Evaluation of the effect of a concurrent chronic total occlusion on long term mortality and left ventricular function in patients after

primary percutaneous intervention. JACC Cardiovasc Interv 2009;2:1128–34.

3. Kirschbaum SW, Baks T, van den Ent M, et al. Evaluation of left ventricular function 3 years after percutaneous coronary intervention of chronic total occlusions. Am J Cardiol 2008;101:179–85.

4. Joyal D, Afilaol J, Rinfret S. Effectiveness of recanalization of chronic total occlusions: a systematic review and meta-analysis. Am Heart J 2011;160:179–87.

5. Grantham JA, Marso SP, Spertus J, et al. Chronic total occlusion angioplasty in the United States. JACC Cardiovasc Interv 2009;2:479–86.

6. Sumitsuji S, Inoue K, Ochiai M, et al. Fundamental wire technique and current standard strategy of percutaneous intervention for chronic total occlusions with histopathologic insights. JACC Cardiovasc Interv 2011;4:941–51.

7. Morino Y, Kimura T, Hayashi Y, et al, J-CTO Registry Investigators. In-hospital outcomes of contemporary percutaneous coronary intervention in patients with chronic total occlusions: insights from the J-CTO registry (multicenter CTO registry in Japan). JACC Cardiovasc Interv 2010;3:143–51.

8. Brilakis ES, Grantham JA, Rinfret S, et al. A percutaneous treatment algorithm for crossing coronary chronic total occlusions. JACC Cardiovasc Interv 2012;5:367–79.

9. Colombo A, Mikhail GW, Michev I, et al. Treating chronic total occlusions using subintimal tracking and reentry: the STAR technique. Catheter Cardiovasc Interv 2005;64:407–11.

10. Carlino M, Godino C, Latib A, et al. Subintimal tracking and re-entry technique with contrast guidance: a safer approach. Catheter Cardiovasc Interv 2008;72:790–6.

11. Whitlow PL, Burke MN, Lombardi WL, et al. Use of a novel crossing and re-entry system in coronary chronic total occlusions that have failed standard crossing techniques: results of the FAST-CTOs trial. JACC Cardiovasc Interv 2012;5:393–401.

12. Lombardi WL. Retrograde PCI: what will they think of next? J Invasive Cardiol 2009;21:543.

13. Whitlow PL, Lombardi WL, Araya M, et al. Initial experience with a dedicated coronary re-entry device for revascularization of chronic total occlusions. Catheter Cardiovasc Interv 2011. [Epub ahead of print].

14. Werner GS, Schofer J, Sievert H, et al. Multicentre experience with the BridgePoint devices to facilitate recanalization of chronic total coronary occlusions through controlled subintimal re-entry. EuroIntervention 2011;7:192–200.

15. Brilakis ES, Lombardi WL, Banerjee S. Use of the Stingray guidewire and the Venture catheter for crossing flush coronary chronic total occlusions due to in-stent restenosis. Catheter Cardiovasc Interv 2010;76:391–4.

Retrograde Dissection and Reentry

Strategies: Common Pitfalls and Troubleshooting

Anja Øksnes, MD[a], Margaret B. McEntegart, MD, PhD[b],*

KEYWORDS

- Chronic total occlusion • Percutaneous coronary intervention • Retrograde • Dissection reentry

KEY POINTS

- The retrograde dissection reentry (RDR) technique is required to treat the most anatomically complex chronic total occlusions (CTOs).
- Pre-procedural planning and thoughtful procedural set-up improves efficiency and success.
- Wire and microcatheter properties should be understood and selected for specific tasks.
- Anticipating pitfalls and developing a knowledge of all the potential solutions improves success and safety.

BACKGROUND

Although contemporary registries report that chronic total occlusion (CTO) percutaneous coronary intervention (PCI) can be performed successfully in more than 80% of patients, this requires the operator to have the skillset to perform the 4 well-described techniques (antegrade wiring [AW], retrograde wiring [RW], antegrade dissection reentry [ADR], retrograde dissection reentry [RDR]), and to be able to use these with a hybrid approach.[1–6] As the complexity of the CTO increases so does the requirement to use dissection reentry techniques (DART) as the primary or bailout strategy.[1–6] Specifically, in the presence of a combination of adverse anatomic characteristics, including an ambiguous proximal cap, occlusion length greater than 20 mm, angulation greater than 45°, a tortuous vessel course, and significant calcification, DART are associated with improved procedural success and safety. Specific indications for RDR over ADR are when the distal cap is located at a bifurcation, the

distal vessel is diffusely diseased and a poor target for antegrade reentry, and when ADR has been unsuccessful. The need to perform RDR correlates with CTO anatomic complexity scores, and is required in approximately one-third of cases with Japanese CTO score ≥3.[1,2]

STRATEGIES

Procedural Planning

Pre-procedural planning including an assessment of patient characteristics, performing detailed angiographic analysis, and developing a hierarchy of strategies has been shown to improve CTO PCI success rates.[2] Coronary computer tomography angiography (CCTA) can be helpful in selected patients.

Patient characteristics

The key characteristics to consider are baseline renal function, left ventricular function, and body habitus.

Although the presence of renal dysfunction limits the safe volume of procedural contrast, a specific advantage of RDR is that the technique

---

[a] Department of Cardiology, Haukeland University Hospital, Jonas Lies vei 65, Bergen 5021, Norway; [b] Department of Cardiology, Golden Jubilee National Hospital, Glasgow G81 4DY, UK
* Corresponding author.
E-mail address: margaret.mcentegart@nhs.net
Twitter: @AnjaKsnes (A.Ø.); @mbmcentegart (M.B.M.)

Intervent Cardiol Clin 10 (2021) 51–64
https://doi.org/10.1016/j.iccl.2020.09.004

necessitates low contrast use. Once a dissection plane has been created, in most situations, further antegrade contrast injections should be avoided to control the size of the sub-intimal space (SIS) and limit hematoma expansion. In addition, the tracking of antegrade and retrograde knuckle wires through the SIS delineates the vessel course without the need for contrast visualization.

Moderate to severe left ventricular systolic dysfunction is associated with some additional risk when using the retrograde approach. Utilization of the collaterals, particularly a single dominant collateral, may induce ischemia and hemodynamic collapse. In the presence of a single dominant collateral, hemodynamic support (intra-aortic balloon pump, Impella, or extracorporeal membrane oxygenation) should be considered, either upfront or as a bailout.[7] Measuring the left ventricular end-diastolic and right heart pressures at the start of the procedure can be helpful to guide this decision making.

Although in contemporary practice radial access is favored in most patients, this is of particular importance in those with a high body mass index (BMI) who are at increased risk of femoral access complications. Distal left radial access can be helpful in this situation to allow pronation of the forearm, which can be rested on the abdomen, facilitating patient and operator comfort. With higher radiation doses anticipated for both the patient and operator, modified angiographic projections and additional radiation projection (eg, Radpads) should be used. A high BMI will accelerate radiation safety thresholds being reached and will limit procedure duration. This may influence your procedural strategy, and specifically in the most complex RDR cases it may be safer to consider a planned investment procedure, with proximal cap modification and collateral exploration, followed by staged completion.

Angiographic analysis

Performing pre-procedural angiographic analysis improves procedural efficiency and success. The anatomic characteristics of the CTO and the available collateral pathways should be assessed to allow a hierarchy of strategies to be devised.

A CTO requiring RDR will usually have several complex anatomic characteristics to consider including an ambiguous or blunt proximal cap, a tortuous or ambiguous vessel course, an occlusion length greater than 20 mm, calcification, a distal cap at a significant bifurcation or with a diseased distal landing zone (**Fig. 1**).

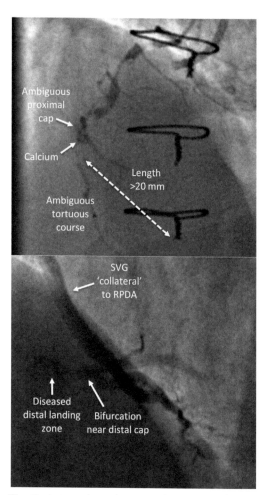

Fig. 1. Antegrade and retrograde angiographic images of RCA CTO with complex anatomic characteristics.

Collateral crossing is essential for retrograde procedural success and therefore the available collateral pathways should be closely studied (**Fig. 2**).[8] The collateral anatomy, including collateral type (septal, epicardial, saphenous vein graft [SVG] or arterial graft), size, tortuosity, and location and angle of exit from the donor vessel and entry to the target vessel, should be assessed to determine their potential utility and any associated hazard (**Fig. 3**). The avoidance of panning during angiography is imperative to assess the course and candidacy of potential interventional collaterals.

Coronary computed tomography angiography

CCTA may provide valuable additional information in pre-procedural planning of CTO PCI.[9] Specifically, for complex occlusions, repeat attempts, and in high risk patients, CCTA may

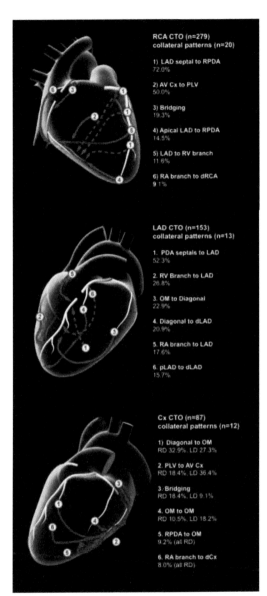

Fig. 2. Prevalence of collateral pathways. AVCx, atrioventricular Cx; Cx, circumflex; dCx, distal Cx; dLAD, distal LAD; dRCA, distal RCA; OM, obtuse marginal; pLAD, proximal LAD; PLV, postero-lateral ventricular; RA, right atrial; RV, right ventricular.

clarify the anatomy, and help predict technical success and procedural risk. Cap ambiguity, occlusion length, vessel course and tortuosity, calcium quantification, and SVG anastomosis location and angulation, can usually be resolved. Fig. 4 shows an example of a proximal right coronary artery (RCA) CTO with an ambiguous proximal cap and vessel course on invasive angiography. The CCTA was performed after an initial PCI attempt resulted in a coronary perforation. With the additional contrast and radiation

exposure, the use of CCTA should be decided on an individual patient basis.

Procedural Set-Up and Equipment
Arterial access and guide catheters
Dual radial access and guide catheters for the target and donor vessels are now routinely used for RDR, especially in the non–post coronary artery bypass graft (CABG) patient. Although most operators use 7 french (Fr), 6 Fr, and 8 Fr (femoral) guides can also be used. A 7 Fr guide can almost always be delivered radially, but if challenging a mother-and-child with a 5 Fr pigtail or multipurpose catheter (110 cm), or the balloon-assisted tracking technique, usually facilitates this. Some scenarios call for oscillating between bypass graft conduits for visualization as well as retrograde options, in which case femoral access may be favorable for adequate guide engagement and support.

The only exceptional situation is when the collaterals are ipsilateral and only one arterial access is available. For the more common situation of ipsilateral collaterals with 2 available arterial access sites "ping-pong" guides should be used. If a single 8-Fr guide has to be used, caution is advised regarding the risk of left main or ostial RCA catheter-induced dissection, and collateral tension and trauma. A single guide also limits the use of adjunctive techniques often required for RDR, including the use of guide extensions or trapping of the retrograde wire to support microcatheter (MC) crossing. In this situation the MC tip-in technique described later is safer.

Support guide catheters should be used for both the target and donor vessels (eg, Extra Back-Up for the left system and Amplatz Left for the RCA). In the target vessel this will facilitate proximal cap penetration and antegrade equipment tracking. In the donor vessel this will provide support for collateral crossing with the MC. A safety workhorse wire should be placed in the donor vessel to maintain luminal access in the event of a catheter-induced dissection.

Guide extensions
The use of an antegrade guide extension in the target vessel improves antegrade support, control of the SIS, and facilitate retrograde reentry and externalization. Once an antegrade dissection plane has been created, the placement of a guide extension reduces antegrade flow into the space, and thus limits SIS expansion and hematoma formation. If available the TrapLiner (Teleflex) guide extension is particularly useful

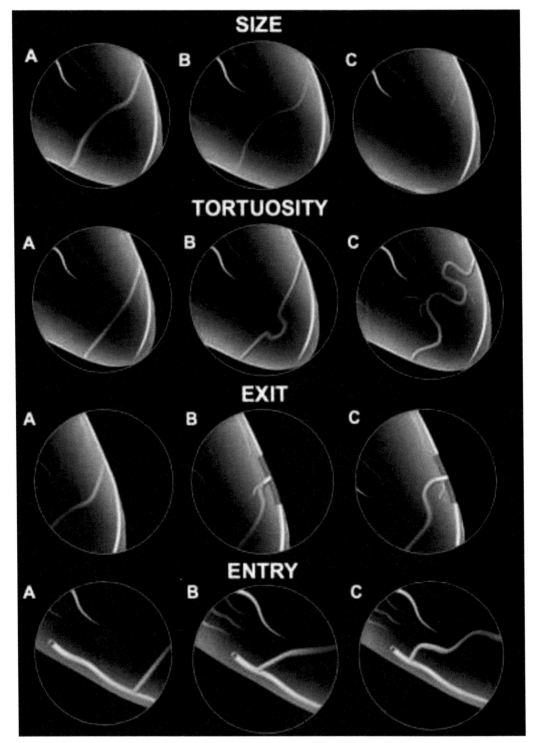

Fig. 3. Collateral anatomy: Size (A) Side-branch like, Collateral Connection 2 (CC2), (B) threadlike connection (CC1), (C) no visible connection (CC0); Tortuosity (A) no acute bends, (B) <2 acute bends, (C) >3 acute bends or bifurcation at acute bend; Exit (A) open angle, (B) acute angle or early bifurcation or stent across exit or proximal vessel tortuosity, (C) any combination or acute angle, bifurcation, stent or proximal tortuosity; Entry (A) Open angle, (B) acute angle or open angle but close to distal cap, (C) acute angle close to distal cap or enters into distal cap.

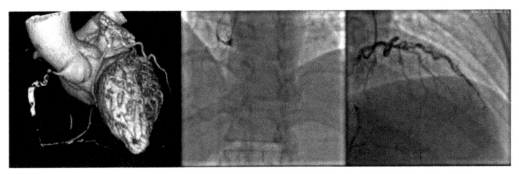

Fig. 4. CCTA and invasive coronary angiography images of RCA CTO: Proximal RCA CTO with ambiguous proximal cap and severe tortuosity revealed by CCTA; CC2 septal collateral from LAD to RPDA also visible on CCTA.

as this also facilitates balloon trapping of over-the-wire equipment, avoiding the need for an accessory trapping balloon or dock extension wire. When performing retrograde reentry, advancing an antegrade guide extension to the planned site of reentry simplifies this maneuver and subsequent externalization, avoiding the need to track the retrograde wire and MC all the way back through the proximal vessel to the antegrade guide catheter (Fig. 5). A guide extension will occasionally be useful retrograde to improve support, particularly when crossing collaterals from the distal right posterior descending artery (RPDA) via a large tortuous RCA, or when using an SVG for retrograde access.

Wires and microcatheters

For RDR, there are dedicated wires to facilitate each of the specific procedural tasks: Proximal

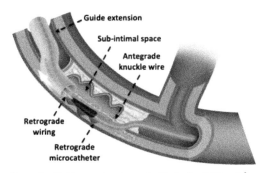

Fig. 5. Guide extension facilitated RDR: After advancing an antegrade knuckle wire, a guide extension is tracked on a balloon to the planned site for reentry; following collateral crossing, the retrograde MC and knuckle wire are advanced to the reentry site; the retrograde knuckle wire is exchanged for a reentry wire, which is advanced into the guide extension. (*Courtesy of* J C Spratt MD FRCP FESC FACC, St. George's, University of London.)

and distal cap crossing, knuckling, collateral crossing, retrograde reentry and wiring, and externalization (Table 1).

Both antegrade and retrograde MCs are required to perform RDR. The MCs available have different crossing profiles and lengths, provide varying degrees of support, and their construction properties dictate how they are optimally tracked, either by sliding, clockwise or anti-clockwise torquing or rapid spinning. Some are often used both antegrade and retrograde, while others are specifically designed to provide increased antegrade support, and others lower profile for crossing small collaterals (Fig. 6).

Dual lumen microcatheters (DLMCs) can be used antegradely to support puncture of a proximal cap if located at a side branch. The Sasuke DLMC (Asahi) can also be used retrogradely to support puncture of the distal cap if located at a bifurcation, but only if the available collateral is large enough to accommodate the larger crossing profile. DLMC are also useful when using an SVG with an acute anastomotic angle, supporting retrograde wire access to the target vessel (Fig. 7).

Procedure Step-by-Step

- Antegrade set-up
  1. Resolving the proximal cap: If unambiguous, the cap can sometimes be punctured with a cap crossing wire and MC; if the proximal cap is ambiguous or uncrossable, there are several potential solutions illustrated in Fig. 8 and discussed later in troubleshooting; if the cap is crossed with the wire but is uncrossable and undilatable with the MC there are several potential options further illustrated in Fig. 9; if the proximal cap is ambiguous and at a side-

Table 1
Retrograde dissection reentry wire properties and tasks

Wire	Tipcoat	Tip load(g)	Polymercoating	Tip Diameter (inch)	Tapered	Wire Tasks		
Fielder XT	Hydrophilic	0,8	Yes	0,009	Yes	Cap Crossing	Reentry and Retrograd Wiring	Knuckling
Fielder XTA	Hydrophilic	1	Yes	0,010	Yes			
Pilot 200	Hydrophilic	4,0	No	0,014	Yes			
Gladius	Hydrophilic	3	Yes	0,014	No			
Gladius MG ES	Hydrophilic	3	Yes	0,014	Yes			
Gaia 2/3/Next	Hydrophilic	3,5/4,5	No	0,011	Yes			
Hornet 14	Hydrophilic	14	No	0,008	Yes			High Penetration wires
Confianza Pro 12	Hydrophilic(tip uncoated)	12	No	0,009	Yes			
Judo 3/6	Hydrophilic	3/6	No	0,008	Yes			
Astato 20/40	Hydrophilic	20/40	No	0,014	Yes			
Halberd	Hydrophilic	12	No	0,014	No			
Miracle Brothers 12	Hydrophobic	13	No	0,014	No			
Sion	Hydrophilic	0,7	No	0,014	No	Collateral Crossing		Epicardial and Septal
SUOH03	Hydrophilic	0,3	No	0,010	No			
Sion Black	Hydrophilic	0,8	Yes	0,014	No			Septal
Fielder XTR	Hydrophilic	0,6	Yes	0,010	Yes			
Samurai RC	Hydrophilic	1,2	No	0,014	No			
Fielder FC	Hydrophilic	0,8	Yes	0,014	No			
R350	Hydrophilic	3	No	0,013	NO	Externalisation		
RG3	Hydrophilic	3	No	0,010	NO			
XT 300	Hydrophilic	0,8	Yes	0,009	Yes			

branch this can sometimes be resolved with an intravascular ultrasound (IVUS) guided puncture.

2. Knuckling: Once the proximal cap has been resolved and crossed a short distance with the MC a knuckle wire should be advanced through the SIS, safely delineating the vessel architecture; if the cap crossing wire and MC have remained within the occlusive plaque a balloon-assisted sub-intimal entry (BASE) may be required to facilitate knuckling; if the knuckle wire cannot be advanced, a power knuckle can be performed. The knuckle wire should be advanced to the planned site for reentry.

- Retrograde set-up
  1. Collateral crossing: A workhorse wire should be placed in the donor vessel; a retrograde MC and workhorse wire with an appropriate tip angle are used to access the collateral, and the wire then exchanged for a collateral crossing wire; for septal collaterals systematic wire surfing is performed supported by the MC, switching between wires as required; for epicardial collaterals controlled wire crossing is performed with a soft-tipped wire with tracking capabilities, usually with the Sion or Suoh 3 (Asahi) supported by a low-profile MC; once the wire accesses the distal target vessel it is followed by the MC, tracking both to the distal cap; a collateral contrast injection via the MC using a 2-mL syringe can be used to further visualize the pathway, but before injecting, ensure blood can be aspirating back. After injecting, clear the contrast with a saline flush, as failure to do so can result in microcatheter failure with increased wire friction.

  2. Resolving the distal cap: The distal cap is usually less resistant and can often be punctured with a cap crossing wire and MC; if the cap is uncrossable or undilatable there are a few potential solutions illustrated in Fig. 10.

  3. Knuckling: Once the distal cap has been crossed a short distance with the retrograde MC, a knuckle wire should be advanced through the SIS, safely delineating the vessel architecture, until overlapping with the antegrade knuckle and MC; the knuckle should be followed by the retrograde MC.

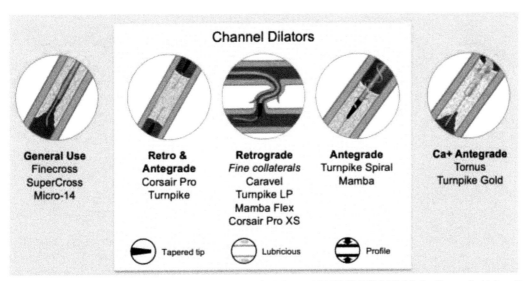

Fig. 6. Microcatheters and their indications. (*Courtesy of* J C Spratt MD FRCP FESC FACC, St. George's, University of London.)

- Reentry
  1. Reentry site: The site of planned reentry should be within the occlusive segment, where both the antegrade and retrograde equipment are definitively within the SIS, and ideally where the knuckle wires are seen to cross or be closest on fluoroscopy; if reentry is unsuccessful, this location can be moved either distally or proximally within the occlusive segment as long as no significant side-branches are crossed; the antegrade MC is trapped out and a guide extension and balloon advanced to the reentry site.
  2. RW: The retrograde knuckle wire is exchanged for a reentry wire; as the antegrade balloon is inflated just beyond the tip of the guide extension

(aiming to connect the antegrade and retrograde SIS), the retrograde wire is aimed at the balloon, advancing it into the guide extension as the balloon deflates; this maneuver may require to be repeated several times until successful; once the retrograde wire has been tracked through the antegrade guide extension into the guide catheter it can be trapped by the retracted antegrade balloon, facilitating tracking of the retrograde MC into the guide extension or catheter.

- Externalization
  1. Wire externalization: With the retrograde MC securely in the antegrade guide catheter or guide extension the antegrade knuckle wire and balloon are removed, and the

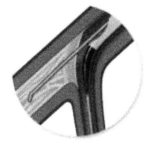

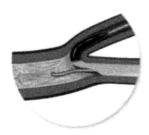

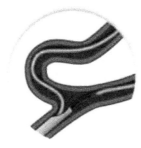

Proximal cap crossing   Distal cap crossing   Retrograde access from graft

Fig. 7. Sasuke dual lumen microcatheter. (*Courtesy of* VP Education, part of the VPMED Group Ltd., Huddersfield, UK; with permission.)

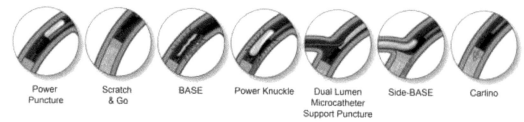

| Power Puncture | Scratch & Go | BASE | Power Knuckle | Dual Lumen Microcatheter Support Puncture | Side-BASE | Carlino |

Fig. 8. Potential solutions for an ambiguous or uncrossable proximal cap.

retrograde wire exchanged for an externalization wire; the wire is advanced through the retrograde MC, all the way through the antegrade guide catheter, and out the Y-connector, facilitated by the wire introducer needle or, if the MC has been advanced into the guide catheter, by retracting the guide extension.

2. Retrograde MC retraction: With the wire externalized, the retrograde MC is retracted to allow equipment to be tracked antegrade to the distal target vessel. Before retracting the MC, the retrograde guide catheter should be disengaged to avoid trauma to the donor vessel; while the MC must remain within the distal target vessel to protect the collateral from possible wire laceration, it needs to be distal enough to avoid interaction with the antegrade equipment and avoid entrapment.

• Procedure completion

1. Lesion preparation, stenting and optimization: Working on the externalized wire provides good support for procedure completion; if there is a bifurcation at the distal cap, an antegrade DLMC can be used to deliver antegrade wires to both branches, with retrieval of the externalized wire as described in the next section; intravascular ultrasound should be used to characterize the occlusive plaque, ensure adequate lesion preparation, and stent optimization.

2. Retrieval of externalized wire: Once the PCI has been completed, the retrograde MC is re-advanced to within the stented segment of the target vessel, allowing the externalized wire to be retrieved without exposing the nonstented vessel or collateral to wire tension; a workhorse collateral safety wire should then be tracked through the retrograde MC into the target vessel and left in place while the retrograde MC is retracted into the donor guide catheter; a retrograde angiogram is performed to check for collateral trauma, with the safety wire facilitating balloon tamponade in the event of a perforation.

Common Pitfalls and Troubleshooting
Uncrossable proximal cap
The proximal cap needs to be resolved no matter what strategy is used to cross the CTO, with the only exception being the minority of cases where the primary strategy is RW. There are several potential solutions to a wire uncrossable proximal cap including (see Fig. 8):

• Increase support: Guide extension; balloon anchoring in a proximal side-branch.

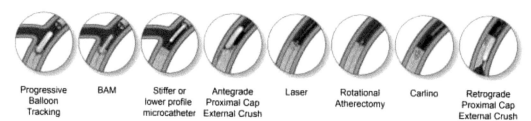

| Progressive Balloon Tracking | BAM | Stiffer or lower profile microcatheter | Antegrade Proximal Cap External Crush | Laser | Rotational Atherectomy | Carlino | Retrograde Proximal Cap External Crush |

Fig. 9. Potential solutions for an undilatable proximal cap. BAM, balloon-assisted micro-dissection.

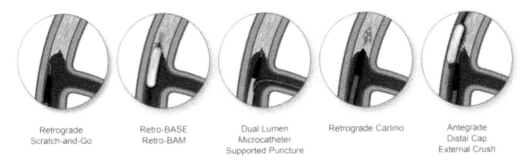

Retrograde   Retro-BASE   Dual Lumen   Retrograde Carlino   Antegrade
Scratch-and-Go   Retro-BAM   Microcatheter   Distal Cap
                                                         Supported Puncture   External Crush

Fig. 10. Potential solutions for an uncrossable or undilatable distal cap. BAM, balloon-assisted micro-dissection.

- Scratch-and-go: A   tapered-tip penetration wire (eg, Confianza Pro 12, Hornet 14, Judo 6) is used to scratch into the vessel wall just proximal to the cap; on feeling resistance the wire should be advanced 1 to 2 mm into the architecture, confirming the wire is moving with the vessel in an orthogonal view; the wire is carefully followed by the tip of the MC and switched for a polymer jacketed wire (eg, Fielder XT/XTA, Pilot 200, Gladius) which is knuckled around the cap while staying in the vessel architecture.
- BASE and power knuckle: An MC is tracked to the proximal cap on a workhorse wire; a second workhorse wire with a non-compliant balloon (NCB) (1:1 size to vessel) is delivered parallel to the MC and inflated to create a dissection; the MC wire is exchanged for a polymer jacketed wire, which, with the NCB retracted and inflated to trap the MC, is knuckled around the cap; after deflating the NCB the MC is advanced over the knuckle wire; this technique may not be feasible if there is only a short segment of vessel proximal to the cap or with ostial occlusions.
- Side-BASE: If there is an ambiguous proximal cap with a side-branch, a semicompliant balloon placed in the side-branch and extending back into main vessel is inflated as a knuckle wire is advanced into the SIS on the opposite side of the vessel; the knuckle wire is tracked around the cap while the balloon protects and blocks the side branch.
- Carlino: A tapered-tip penetration wire is embedded into the proximal cap, followed by the tip of the MC. Using a 2-mL syringe a small volume of contrast is forced into cap to create a hydraulic dissection and weaken the cap. A polymer jacketed wire is then knuckled into the SIS.
- Increased penetration MC: Turnpike Spiral, Turnpike Gold, or Tornus.
- Antegrade external cap crush: When a knuckle wire has been tracked beside the proximal cap but is unable to progress, balloon dilatation on this wire can externally crush and weaken the cap, then allowing a parallel MC and wire to progress.
- Rotational or laser atherectomy.
- Retrograde external cap crush: A retrograde knuckle wire is tracked past the proximal cap. The retrograde MC is exchanged for a long low-profile balloon, which is advanced into the SIS beside the proximal cap and inflated to externally crush the cap, then allowing the antegrade MC and wire to progress.

Collateral crossing

Collaterals with the potential to be used for retrograde access are present in 64% of CTOs.[8] The most common failure mode with the retrograde approach is the inability to cross the collaterals with a wire or MC, with contemporary registries reporting approximately 20% of collaterals attempted are uncrossable.[10] The most commonly used collaterals are septals, followed by epicardials, and then bypass grafts. For each collateral type, the approach and associated risks are different.

Septal crossing: If collaterals are uncrossable with the initial wire choice, alternatives with different properties should be considered (eg, Sion, Sion Black, Suoh-3, Fielder XTR, Samurai RC); If a collateral is crossed with the wire but uncrossable with the MC there are several potential solutions, including the following:

- Increase retrograde support: Guide extension; donor system anchoring in side-branch or stented segment; switching to an 8-Fr femoral guide or 7.5-Fr radial sheathless guide.

- Septal collateral balloon dilatation: Using a low-profile long balloon (eg, 1.0, 1.2, or 1.5 × 20).
- Change for a lower profile or new 150 cm MC (MC fatigue): Caravel, Turnpike LP, Mamba Flex, Corsair Pro XS.
- Use a short MC: Use the increased torque and push to dilate the channel, then switch back to a 150-cm MC.
- Trap the retrograde wire with an antegrade balloon: Increasing support to deliver the retrograde MC.
- Exchange septal crossing wire for a more supportive wire: Sion Black or Fielder FC.
- Explore a different septal or other available collateral.
- Switch to an antegrade strategy (ADR): Leaving retrograde marker wire.

Epicardial crossing: This is a significantly higher risk technique requiring a different and more cautious approach; epicardial collaterals are more fragile with a higher risk of perforation; soft crossing wires (eg, Sion, Suoh 3) and MC (Caravel, Turnpike LP, Finecross) should be used; there is often dynamic motion and limited control of the wire and MC on the epicardial surface of the heart with an associated risk of collateral trauma. If unable to follow the wire with the MC, unlike in septal collaterals, balloon dilatation should not be performed.

SVG crossing: In patients post CABG, SVGs can be efficient and safe conduits for retrograde access; although easiest through a patent graft with minimal degeneration, diseased or occluded grafts can also be used; other anatomic considerations are the location and angle of the graft anastomosis to the target vessel to facilitate retrograde tracking to the distal cap (Fig. 11); optimizing retrograde support with an Amplatz left or Multipurpose guide and guide extension is key to performing RDR via an SVG; a workhorse safety wire should be placed into the distal target vessel; a parallel 150 cm MC and wire (eg, Sion, Sion Black, Gladius, Pilot 200) are then tracked across the graft anastomosis and retrogradely to the distal cap.

If RW from the SVG is not possible, there are a number of potential solutions:

- Exchange for a different wire.
- Track a DLMC on the safety wire to the site of the graft anastomosis: Increasing support for RW (see Fig. 7).

- Track a blocking balloon on the safety wire and inflate in the distal vessel just beyond the graft anastomosis: Allows deflection of the second wire retrogradely.

If the wire tracks retrograde to the target vessel but the MC is unable to follow there are a number of potential solutions:

- Exchange for a lower profile MC: Caravel or Turnpike LP.
- Use a more supportive retrograde wire: Gladius or Pilot 200.
- Balloon dilate the anastomosis: On the retrograde wire with a small low-profile balloon, or if not possible balloon antegradely on the safety wire, to modify fibrotic tissue at the graft insertion site.
- Trap the retrograde wire with an antegrade balloon: Increasing support for delivery of the retrograde MC.
- Perform a retrograde Carlino at the anastomosis: To clarify anatomic ambiguity and weaken any resistant tissue.

Internal mammary artery (IMA) grafts: Should be used only for retrograde access if all other options have been exhausted and there is no antegrade solution. Anatomic characteristics including graft tortuosity, angle and location of graft anastomosis relative to the septal collaterals (for RCA target vessels) need to be considered to determine the potential utility and safety of this approach (Fig. 12); a safety wire from the IMA to distal left anterior descending (LAD) is essential. The troubleshooting discussed previously for SVG retrograde access also applies for the IMA and another important factor is the length of the retrograde pathway, particularly if using the IMA to access the RCA retrogradely via the LAD septals. Using 80-cm to 90-cm guide catheters with guide extensions will avoid issues with reach between the antegrade and retrograde systems. Using the IMA to access a dominant collateral (eg, LAD to RPDA) increases the risk of ischemia and potentially hemodynamic collapse, thus insertion of upfront 5-Fr femoral access to facilitate rapid delivery of mechanical circulatory support may be considered in patients with low reserve.

Uncrossable distal cap

The distal cap is usually less resistant than the proximal cap, being exposed to the lower pressure of the collateral circulation. An uncrossable

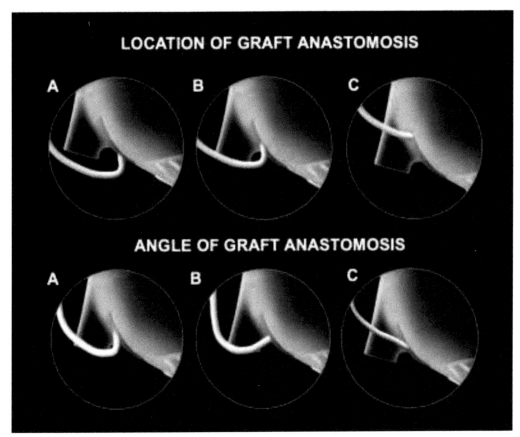

Fig. 11. SVG anatomy and retrograde access: Location of graft anastomosis (*A*) >10 mm from distal cap, (*B*) <10 mm from distal cap, (*C*) At distal cap; Angle of graft anastomosis (*A*) >90°, (*B*) 45° to 90°, (*C*) <45°.

distal cap is therefore more commonly encountered post CABG where the distal cap is exposed to near aortic pressure. There are several potential solutions, including the following:

- Increase retrograde support: Guide extension; donor system anchoring.
- Retrograde scratch-and-go.
- Retrograde Carlino.
- Supportive retrograde MC: Turnpike Spiral 150.
- Retrograde DLMC: If the distal cap is at a bifurcation and the septal collateral large enough to allow tracking this increases support for distal cap crossing (see Fig. 7).
- Antegrade external cap crush: After advancing an antegrade knuckle wire in the SIS to beyond the distal cap, balloon dilatation externally crushes and weaken the distal cap, then allowing the retrograde MC to progress (see Fig. 10).

Unable to connect the antegrade and retrograde spaces

If initial attempts, as described earlier, to connect the antegrade and retrograde SIS are unsuccessful, simply retracting the balloon into the guide extension creating more space will often allow wire reentry. If still unsuccessful there are several potential solutions:

- Use a larger antegrade balloon to expand and connect the SIS.
- Use a higher penetration force retrograde reentry wire: Confianza Pro 12, Hornet 14, Astato 20.
- Reknuckle antegradely or retrogradely to ensure both wires are in the SIS.
- IVUS to check that both wires are in the SIS and confirm 1:1 balloon:vessel sizing.
- Move the site of reentry proximal or distal: Staying within the segment where you know both wires are in the SIS.
- Switch to the controlled antegrade reentry technique (CART): Exchange the

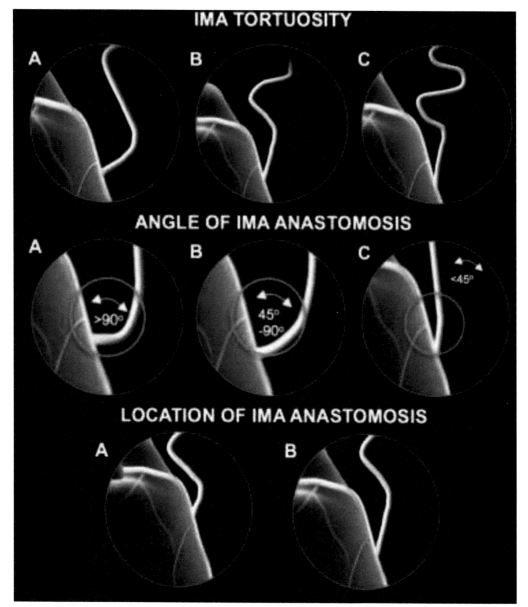

Fig. 12. IMA anatomy and retrograde access: Tortuosity (A) mild, (B) moderate, (C) severe; Angle of graft anastomosis (A) >90°, (B) 45° to 90°, (C) <45°; Location of graft anastomosis (A) proximal to septal collateral, (B) distal to septal collateral.

antegrade balloon and knuckle wire for an MC and reentry wire (eg, Gladius, Pilot 200, Gaia 3rd); exchange the retrograde MC for a long retrograde balloon; while inflating and deflating the retrograde balloon aim the antegrade reentry wire toward it, reentering the distal true lumen.

Retrograde microcatheter unable to track through the occlusive segment
If after retrograde reentry you are unable to follow the wire with the retrograde MC, there are several potential solutions:

- Trap the retrograde wire within the guide or guide extension with the antegrade balloon.
- Advance the antegrade guide extension to capture the retrograde MC.
- Exchange for a new retrograde MC (MC fatigue).
- Exchange the retrograde wire for a more supportive wire.
- Increase retrograde support: Guide extension, donor vessel anchoring.
- Supportive retrograde MC: Turnpike Spiral 150

- Rendezvous/tip-in MC technique: Wiring the antegrade MC with the retrograde wire (within the guide or guide extension); then advance the antegrade MC over retrograde wire as the retrograde MC is slowly retracted.
- Modify the resistant segment with an antegrade balloon.
- Dilate retrogradely with a long low-profile balloon.
- Switch to CART.

Externalization

Wire externalization is sometimes difficult or not possible due to extreme resistance in the guide and MC system. There are a few potential solutions:

- Use an alternative dedicated externalization wire.
- Use a 300 cm CTO wire: Fielder XTA or Fielder FC.
- Use the rendezvous/tip-in technique: Wiring the retrograde MC with an antegrade wire and then advancing the antegrade MC as the retrograde MC is gradually retracted; usually easiest at a curve in the guide catheter where both MCs hug the outer curvature.

Occasionally, it is not possible to wire the antegrade guide catheter with the retrograde wire. In this situation, snaring of the externalization wire in the aorta can be performed:

- Snaring: The retrograde wire and MC should be advanced into the aortic root and the wire exchanged for a dedicated externalization wire; all antegrade equipment is removed and the guide catheter retracted to the aortic arch; an Ensnare 18 × 30-mm tulip snare should be advanced through the antegrade guide out into the aortic arch; the snare can be spun while simultaneously advancing the externalization wire back and forward until it is successfully captured and can be retracted into the antegrade guide; as the snared wire is pulled back through the antegrade guide, the guide is advanced to reengage the target vessel; the donor guide catheter should be disengaged to avoid trauma; on retrieving the snared wire from the guide the back-end requires to be cut off to allow antegrade equipment to be tracked.

Occasionally, ischemia or hemodynamic compromise will require the retrograde system to be removed before procedure completion:

- Early retrieval of the externalized wire: An antegrade MC is tracked on the externalized wire to a straight segment of the distal vessel, carefully keeping a short distance between the tips of the MCs; the externalized wire is slowly retracted through the retrograde system; an antegrade workhorse wire is delivered and used to complete the procedure; alternatively this can be done using an antegrade DLMC allowing the delivery of an antegrade wire before the externalized wire being retrieved.

In addition to the solutions described previously for RDR, the comprehensive paper by Riley and colleagues[11] provides troubleshooting algorithms for all CTO PCI techniques.

Complications

The complication rates in retrograde CTO PCI are higher than with the antegrade approach, due to both the more complex anatomy and risks associated with collateral crossing.[12] This includes higher risks of perforation and tamponade, peri-procedural myocardial infarction, access site complications, stroke, acute kidney injury, and radiation skin damage.

The CTO operator should be trained in the avoidance and management of these complications:

Perforations

- An emergency trolley with a pericardiocentesis kit, coils, thrombin, covered stents, and an echo machine, should be kept in the catheterization laboratory.
- Septal collateral: Usually benign, but monitor for septal hematoma, which can cause hemodynamic compromise due to impaired ventricular filling. Distal septals may at times take an epicardial course and can rarely cause tamponade.
- Epicardial collateral: Block both antegrade and retrograde entry with coils, fat, thrombin, or covered stents.
- Main vessel: Immediately inflate a balloon across the perforation; may require covered stent delivery with ping-pong guide catheter.

Access site

- Use biradial access if feasible.
- For femoral access perform ultrasound and fluoroscopic-guided puncture.

Donor vessel dissection

- Always place a safety workhorse wire in the donor vessel.
- Back out the donor guide when retrieving retrograde equipment.

Donor vessel thrombosis

- Maintain activated clotting time greater than 350 and monitor every 20 minutes.

SUMMARY

The anatomically most complex CTOs can be resolved only with the RDR technique. This is therefore an essential skillset for the CTO operator aiming to consistently achieve CTO PCI success rates greater than 80%. There are many pitfalls with this technique, and the ability to systematically troubleshoot is a mindset that can be developed with experience. The retrograde approach is known to be associated with higher complication rates, and therefore alternative antegrade techniques should always be considered, and the appropriateness and risk-benefit balance of the procedure discuss with each individual patient.

CLINICS CARE POINTS

- Appropriate patient selection and informed consent is essential before proceeding with these complex high-risk procedures.
- The CTO operator requires training in each of the sequential steps of the RDR technique, and to have knowledge of the troubleshooting options for each of these steps.
- An understanding of how to avoid and manage all potential complications is key to minimising patient hazard.

DISCLOSURE

M.B. McEntegart has proctorship agreement with Boston Scientific. A. Øksnes nothing to disclose.

REFERENCES

1. Wilson WM, Walsh SJ, Yan AT, et al. Hybrid approach improves success of chronic total occlusion angioplasty. Heart 2016;102:1486–93.
2. Maeremans J, Walsh S, Knaapen P, et al. The hybrid algorithm for treating chronic total occlusions in Europe: the RECHARGE Registry. J Am Coll Cardiol 2016;68:1958–70.
3. Tajti P, Karmpaliotis D, Alaswad K, et al. The hybrid approach to chronic total occlusion percutaneous coronary intervention: update from the PROGRESS CTO Registry. JACC Cardiovasc Interv 2018;11:1325–35.
4. Sapontis J, Salisbury AC, Yeh RW, et al. Early procedural and health status outcomes after chronic total occlusion angioplasty: a report from the OPEN-CTO Registry (Outcomes, Patient Health Status, and Efficiency in Chronic Total Occlusion Hybrid Procedures). JACC Cardiovasc Interv 2017;10:1523–34.
5. Konstantinidis NV, Werner GS, Deftereos S, et al. Temporal trends in chronic total occlusion interventions in Europe. Circ Cardiovasc Interv 2018;11:e006229.
6. Wu EB, Tsuchikane E, Ge L, et al. Retrograde versus antegrade approach for coronary chronic total occlusion in an algorithm-driven contemporary asia-pacific multicenter registry: comparison of outcomes. Heart Lung Circ 2019;28:1490–500.
7. Riley RF, McCabe JM, Kalra S, et al. Impella-assisted chronic total occlusion percutaneous coronary interventions: a multicenter retrospective analysis. Catheter Cardiovasc Interv 2018;92:1261–7.
8. Opolski MP, Achenbach S. CT angiography for revascularization of CTO: crossing the borders of diagnosis and treatment. JACC Cardiovasc Imaging 2015;8:846–58.
9. McEntegart MB, Badar AA, Ahmad FA, et al. The collateral circulation of coronary chronic total occlusions. EuroIntervention 2016;11:e1596–603.
10. Yamane M, Muto M, Matsubara T, et al. Contemporary retrograde approach for the recanalisation of coronary chronic total occlusion: on behalf of the Japanese Retrograde Summit Group. EuroIntervention 2013;9:102–9.
11. Riley RF, Walsh SJ, Kirtane AJ, et al. Algorithmic solutions to common problems encountered during chronic total occlusion angioplasty: the algorithms within the algorithm. Catheter Cardiovasc Interv 2019;93:286–97.
12. Megaly M, Ali A, Saad M, et al. Outcomes with retrograde versus antegrade chronic total occlusion revascularization. Catheter Cardiovasc Interv 2019. https://doi.org/10.1002/ccd.28616.

Subintimal Plaque Modification and Subintimal Dissection and Reentry
Strategies to Turn Failure into Success

Michael Megaly, MD, MS, Ashish Pershad, MD, MS*

KEYWORDS

- Chronic total occlusion • Subintimal plaque modification • SPM • CTO

KEY POINTS

- Ultimately successful chronic total occlusion percutaneous coronary intervention (CTO PCI) when traditional antegrade and retrograde techniques fail depends, in large part, on the ability to perform bailout strategies involving subintimal plaque modification.
- Subintimal tracking and reentry technique in which an intentional dissection is created using a knuckled wire distal to CTO to reenter the true lumen, followed by balloon angioplasty with an intent to achieve TIMI III flow. In modern practice, stenting is deferred and CTO PCI reattempted at CTO PCI after 2 to 3 months to allow for healing of dissection planes and reassessment of flow.
- Limited data on subintimal plaque modification have shown good outcomes with 70% vessel patency at follow-up and no increased risk of periprocedural complications.

 Video content accompanies this article at http://www.interventional.theclinics.com.

INTRODUCTION

Chronic total occlusion (CTO) percutaneous coronary intervention (PCI) has evolved over the last decade. The updated hybrid algorithm, advancement in retrograde techniques and equipment, and dissemination of antegrade dissection and reentry techniques (ADR) have played an essential role in this evolution. There is a disconnect between the outcomes in self-reported registries and national databases such as the National Cardiovascular Data Registry (NCDR). Attempt rates, as well as procedural success rates, are 20% points lower in the NCDR registry when compared with outcomes in published CTO trials with expert operators.[1–3] When CTO recanalization with traditional techniques such as antegrade/retrograde wire

escalation or antegrade/retrograde dissection reentry is not achievable, the concept of subintimal tracking and reentry (STAR) is used. Subintimal plaque modification (SPM) and its different iterations are useful.

The concept of plaque modification and healing of dissections is not unique to CTO PCI. Spontaneous coronary artery dissections and iatrogenic dissections in non-CTO vessels have a propensity to heal if flow in the vessel is restored and there is no untreated angiographic stenosis.[4–6]

DISCUSSION

The Original Subintimal Tracking and Reentry Technique

The STAR technique was introduced in 2005 by Colombo and colleagues.[7] The STAR technique

---

Funding: None.
University of Arizona College of Medicine Phoenix, 475 North 5th Street, Phoenix, AZ 85004, USA
* Corresponding author.
E-mail address: apershad@email.arizona.edu

is an antegrade dissection and reentry technique. It is performed by using a stiff guidewire to create a subintimal dissection flap. This guidewire is then exchanged for a polymer-jacketed guidewire, configured as an umbrella handle, within a microcatheter. The guidewire is pushed to form a knuckle within the subintimal space with unpredictable, spontaneous reentry into the true lumen, usually at a bifurcation. Although technical success rates were high, the STAR technique depends on creating a subintimal channel with the loss of many side branches and often poor runoff. The poor distal runoff and the long zone of subintimal stenting led to high rates of restenosis and reocclusion.[8] This technique was independently associated with the risk of reocclusion (odds ratio [OR]: 29.5; $P<.001$).[9] Because of the high rates of restenosis and reocclusion, STAR has been relegated as a last resort strategy in contemporary CTO PCI.

The Modified Subintimal Tracking and Reentry Techniques
Multiple iterations of the original STAR technique have been proposed.

Contrast-enhanced subintimal tracking and reentry
The contrast-enhanced STAR is one such iteration.[8] This technique depends on creating a contrast-enhanced dissection plane by intentional injection of 2 to 3 cc of contrast after crossing the proximal cap of the CTO. Three potential outcomes are possible after injecting contrast past the proximal cap: (1) creation of a tubular dissection outlining the vessel course with distal true lumen visualization, which could then be reached with antegrade CTO wiring techniques; (2) creation of a "storm cloud" dissection implying penetration of contrast into the adventitia posing a higher risk for perforation and no distal true lumen visualization; and (3) microchannel visualization allowing for crossing the CTO with soft polymeric low-gram force wires without a notable dissection, making intraplaque antegrade wiring feasible. The MACE rates and perforation rates, although high with contrast-enhanced STAR, were lower than that reported with the original STAR technique.[8]

Mini-subintimal tracking and reentry
In 2012, Galassi and colleagues introduced the concept of the mini-STAR technique that depends on minimizing the subintimal dissection plane by using a special configuration forming 2 small curves 1 to 2 mm and 3 to 5 mm from the tip of a Fielder XT wire (Asahi Intecc, Nagoya, Japan).[10] This guidewire has a low tip load and a hybrid coating (SLIP over tip and PTFE over shaft) as well as a 3-cm "transition zone" between the shaft and the soft tip allowing the formation of a smaller knuckle that is easier to navigate than the Pilot family or Whisper wire used in the original STAR case series. The smaller knuckle, along with the softer tip, minimizes the subintimal hematoma extension and allows for possible reentry closer to the distal cap rather than when reentry is performed with stiffer jacketed wires. Long-term follow-up of 117 patients treated with the mini-STAR technique showed that restenosis and reocclusion rates were still high at 25% and 12.5%, respectively, making this another potential bailout strategy but not suitable as a primary strategy for CTO recanalization.[11]

Subintimal plaque modification
Subintimal plaque modification is defined as balloon angioplasty of the subintimal space within the CTO body and occasionally beyond the distal cap of the CTO with a balloon sized 1:1 to the vessel diameter or greater than 2 mm in diameter to increase chances of TIMI 3 antegrade flow. It is performed in cases of technical failure or imminent failure during CTO PCI when access to the distal true lumen is not feasible. Stenting of the subintimal space is deferred during this phase of the procedure. Definitive treatment with drug-eluting stents is performed in 2 to 3 months after this "investment procedure" to allow for possible healing of dissection planes and resolution of hematoma. Studies that have reported the use of SPM[12–17] are summarized in Table 1.

Clinical Outcomes with Subintimal Plaque Modification
There is a benefit in the patient-reported health status outcomes with SPM. In the OPEN-CTO registry (Outcomes, Patient Health Status, and Efficiency in Chronic Total Occlusion) SPM was performed in 59 (42.8%) of 138 patients who had failed CTO PCI.[13] One-month health status follow-up measured by the coronary artery disease (CAD)-specific Seattle Angina Questionnaire (SAQ-SS) was significantly better in patients who had SPM compared with those who did not. The delta in the SAQ-SS was 28.3 ± 21.7 in the patients who underwent SPM compared with 16.8 ± 20.2 in the group that did not undergo SPM and had a failed CTO PCI ($P = 0.012$). The SAQ anginal frequency score, as well as the SAQ quality of

Table 1
Summary of the studies reporting the use of subintimal plaque modification

Study	Years	Number of Cases	Target Vessel	J-CTO Score	Time to Repeat Procedure	Success Rate	Complications	Comments
Wilson et al,[16] 2013	-	4	RCA (75%) LAD (25%)	Not mentioned	1.5–4 mo	100%	-	Four case reports
Visconti et al,[14] 2015	January 2010 to June 2012	69 (patients had successful STAR but with delayed stenting)	RCA (46%) LCx (42%) LAD (12%)	Not mentioned	2.5 ± 0.3 mo	Total (94.2%) 79.7% at the first reattempt 14.5% at the second reattempt	Perforation (2.5%) Cardiac tamponade (1.4%) Pericardiocentesis (1.4%) Periprocedural MI (increase in troponin I >5 times above the ULN) (55%)	Patients were compared with a historical cohort of immediate stenting after STAR technique (60 patients). SPM was associated with shorter dissection and stent length at 3-mo follow-up. The risk of stent thrombosis, myocardial infarction, and death was significantly lower in the SPM group at 6 mo

(continued on next page)

Study	Years	Number of Cases	Target Vessel	J-CTO Score	Time to Repeat Procedure	Success Rate	Complications	Comments
Wilson et al,[15] 2016	January 2012 to December 2014	151	Not mentioned	Mean ± SD (3.1 ± 1.2)	3 (IQR 1.8–4.3) mo	96% at repeat attempt	Not mentioned	SPM was performed in 62% of cases at the end of the unsuccessful first procedure. This increased the chance of subsequent success (96% vs 71%) compared with those who did not have an investment procedure
Hirai et al,[13] 2018	January 2014 to July 2015	59	RCA (64.4%) LCx (18.6%) LAD (15.3%) LM (1.7%)	40.7% had J-CTO score of 3 or higher	No repeat procedure.	No repeat procedure	Perforation (10.2%) Acute MI (1.7%) Emergent surgery (1.7%) In-hospital death (1.7%)	SPM was performed in 59 patients (42.8%) of patients who had failed CTO PCI in the OPEN CTO registry (138) One-mo health status follow-up by CAD-specific SAQ was significantly better in patients who had SPM compared with those who did not

Goleski et al,[12] 2019	January 2015 to May 2017	32 (deferred stenting after STAR)	RCA (50%) LCx (44%) LAD (6%)	Median [IQR] (2.5 [1–3])	2.4 (IQR 1.7–3.3) mo	88%	Up to 30 d after the procedure Perforation (3%) Acute MI (3%) Stent thrombosis (3%)	SPM was performed in 45 patients (5.8%) of patients who underwent CTO PCI (781), but only 32 (4.1%) patients had repeat procedure
Xenogiannis et al,[17] 2019	January 2012 to January 2019	57	RCA (50%) LCx (29%) LAD (21%)	Mean ± SD (3.2 ± 1.1)	60 (IQR 49, 90) d	83%	Perforation (1.7%) Pericardiocentesis (1.7%) Acute MI (1.7%)	SPM was used in 119 patients (13%) who had failed prior attempts (935)

Abbreviations: CTO, chronic total occlusion; IQR, interquartile range; J-CTO, Japanese chronic total occlusion score; LAD, left anterior descending artery; LCx, left circumflex artery; MI, myocardial infarction; RCA, right coronary artery; SPM, subintimal plaque modification; STAR, subintimal tracking and reentry; ULN, upper limits of normal.

life scores, were higher in the group that underwent SPM as compared with the group that did not undergo SPM, although these did not achieve statistical significance. The observation that restoration of antegrade TIMI flow in the CTO vessel after SPM is the sole predictor of vessel patency on follow-up angiography makes it unlikely that a placebo effect, regression to the mean, and adjustment of activity level or antianginal medications were responsible for the improvement in the patient-reported outcomes.

In the PROGRESS CTO registry, SPM was performed slightly more often in 13% of patients who had failed prior attempts. They identified waiting for at least 2 months between the index and definitive procedure as a predictor for improved technical success (94% vs 69%, $P = .015$).[17]

Technical Pearls of Subintimal Plaque Modification

1 The recognition of futility and going into failure mode is the signal to the operator to consider bailout strategies of which SPM is the most favored.
2 Understanding the mechanism of failure helps set up the base for SPM, for example, failure of ADR with the Stingray balloon beyond the distal cap, and allows for swapping out the Stingray balloon with a microcatheter and then using a dedicated knuckle wire such as the Fielder XT (ASAHI Intecc, Japan), Mongo Gladius (ASAHI Intecc, Japan), Pilot 200 (Abbott Vascular, USA), or Bandit (Teleflex, USA) to perform an STAR procedure. This is then followed by angioplasty of the CTO body and beyond the distal cap completing the SPM procedure with the restoration of antegrade flow.
3 Deferral of stenting: one of the essential aspects of SPM is deferral of stenting during the index procedure. This is a difficult concept to grasp for operators and staff alike. Allowing dissection planes to heal and hematomas to shrink will reduce the need for stents on the subsequent attempt and preserve more side branches.
4 Timing of reattempt: consensus about reattempt timing is lacking, but it is suggested that a minimum of 8 weeks be given for dissections and hematomas to heal. Clinical symptoms often dictate the timing for a reattempt.

A step-by-step approach to SPM is shown in Fig. 1 and a case example (Videos 1–6).

Complications and Concerns of Subintimal Plaque Modification

Although the safety of the procedure has been demonstrated in the small studies published to date,[12–17] with the risk of perforation and MACE similar to the overall risk in CTO PCI procedures and even lower than unsuccessful CTO PCI in some series,[13] larger-scale studies are required to define its safety better.

Modern Approach to Subintimal Tracking and Reentry

When approaching a CTO with antegrade wire escalation, targeted antegrade re-entry, and retrograde approaches are unsuccessful then the use of STAR as a bailout can be highly effective. In the modern approach STAR is performed with soft polymeric wires that make smaller knuckles. Mongo, Fielder XT-R, and Fighter are effective. The operator should look for the wire to shrink and accelerate in the distal vessel as the point of reentry; then using 2.0 to 2.5 diameter balloons the distal vessel should be dilated and the more proximal vessel with larger balloons. Antegrade injections can be taken at this point to evaluate for TIMI III flow and what branches need to be rescued. It is recommended to use STAR for as many of the major outflow branches as possible. To be able to do so the operator should be facile with wire redirect and knuckle redirect techniques to rescue as many side branches that are deemed clinically relevant. Delayed stenting is then prefered at 8 to 12 weeks. Recent data have shown that more than 50% of STAR will return open and need just a workhorse wire and stenting. Of the remainder that have reoccluded repeat attempts have a 90% success rate.

SUMMARY AND FUTURE DIRECTIVES

One of the challenges with STAR has been the 50% of cases in which after STAR, the vessel remains occluded or is found to have reoccluded on angiography 3 months after the investment procedure. This event is not unexpected, and the reattempt success rate should be higher than 90% at this procedure as the anatomy and architecture have been changed by the original procedure. The therapeutic goal after STAR should, therefore, be the establishing of TIMI-3 flow in the CTO vessel. Visconti and colleagues observed that the presence of moderate-to-severe spontaneous echo contrast in the nonoccluded dissected segment on intravascular ultrasound was associated with early reocclusion.[14] Spontaneous echo contrast is a surrogate

Subintimal Plaque modification step-by-step

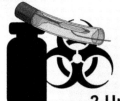

1-Recognition of technical failure or imminent failure

2-Understand the mechanism of failure (eg, failure of antegrade reentry)

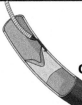

3- Use a knuckle wire (eg, gladius mongo) through a microcatheter to create dissection distal to CTO (STAR)

4-Balloon angioplasty with 1:1 sizing

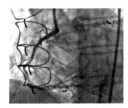

5-Ensure TIMI III flow

6-Avoid stenting

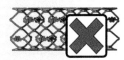

7-Re-attemt after a minimum of 2–3 mo

Fig. 1. A step-by-step approach to subintimal plaque modification.

for slow flow and its presence makes it unlikely that the vessel will remain open. Another intriguing concept is the combination of drug-eluting balloons with noncompliant balloons during the investment procedure. The theory being that the drug-eluting balloon would potentially reduce neointimal hyperplasia while maintaining TIMI 3 flow through the fenestrations of the dissection planes.[18] Longer follow-up of a larger number of patients will help further clarify the role of SPM in contemporary CTO PCI.

CLINICS CARE POINTS

- SPM is a valuable skill set when CTO PCI is imminently unsuccessful using traditional techniques like antegrade wiring, antegrade dissection re-entry and retrograde dissection reentry.
- Angioplasty with an adequately sized balloon of the occluded segment and deferral of stenting are the tenets of SPM.
- Reattempt of the CTO at 8-12 weeks lead to secondary success rates of >90%.
- The role of drug eluting balloons in the context of SPM is an intriguing concept warranting further clinical research.

DISCLOSURES

The authors have no conflicts of interest to disclose.

SUPPLEMENTARY DATA

Supplementary data related to this article can be found online at 10.1016/j.iccl.2020.09.012.

REFERENCES

1. Tajti P, Burke MN, Karmpaliotis D, et al. Update in the percutaneous management of coronary chronic total occlusions. JACC Cardiovasc Interventions 2018;11(7):615–25.
2. Sapontis J, Salisbury AC, Yeh RW, et al. Early procedural and health status outcomes after chronic total occlusion angioplasty: a report from the OPEN-CTO registry (Outcomes, patient health status, and efficiency in chronic total occlusion hybrid procedures). JACC Cardiovasc Interventions 2017;10(15):1523–34.
3. Serruys P, Hamburger J, Fajadet J, et al. Total occlusion trial with angioplasty by using laser guidewire. The TOTAL trial. Eur Heart J 2000;21(21):1797–805.
4. Alfonso F, Paulo M, Lennie V, et al. Spontaneous coronary artery dissection: long-term follow-up of a large series of patients prospectively managed with a "conservative" therapeutic strategy. JACC Cardiovasc Interventions 2012;5(10):1062–70.
5. Tweet MS, Hayes SN, Pitta SR, et al. Clinical features, management, and prognosis of spontaneous coronary artery dissection. Circulation 2012;126(5):579–88.
6. Mortensen KH, Thuesen L, Kristensen IB, et al. Spontaneous coronary artery dissection: a Western Denmark Heart Registry study. Catheter Cardiovasc Interv 2009;74(5):710–7.
7. Colombo A, Mikhail GW, Michev I, et al. Treating chronic total occlusions using subintimal tracking and reentry: the STAR technique. Catheter Cardiovasc Interv 2005;64(4):407–11 [discussion: 412].
8. Carlino M, Godino C, Latib A, et al. Subintimal tracking and reentry technique with contrast guidance: a safer approach. Catheter Cardiovasc Interv 2008;72(6):790–6.
9. Valenti R, Vergara R, Migliorini A, et al. Predictors of reocclusion after successful drug-eluting stent-supported percutaneous coronary intervention of chronic total occlusion. J Am Coll Cardiol 2013;61(5):545–50.
10. Galassi AR, Tomasello SD, Costanzo L, et al. Mini-STAR as bailout strategy for percutaneous coronary intervention of chronic total occlusion. Catheter Cardiovasc Interv 2012;79(1):30–40.
11. Galassi AR, Boukhris M, Tomasello SD, et al. Long-term clinical and angiographic outcomes of the mini-STAR technique as a bailout strategy for percutaneous coronary intervention of chronic total occlusion. Can J Cardiol 2014;30(11):1400–6.
12. Goleski PJ, Nakamura K, Liebeskind E, et al. Revascularization of coronary chronic total occlusions with subintimal tracking and reentry followed by deferred stenting: experience from a high-volume referral center. Catheter Cardiovasc Interv 2019;93(2):191–8.
13. Hirai T, Grantham JA, Sapontis J, et al. Impact of subintimal plaque modification procedures on health status after unsuccessful chronic total occlusion angioplasty. Catheter Cardiovasc Interv 2018;91(6):1035–42.
14. Visconti G, Focaccio A, Donahue M, et al. Elective versus deferred stenting following subintimal recanalization of coronary chronic total occlusions. Catheter Cardiovasc Interv 2015;85(3):382–90.
15. Wilson W, Walsh S, Yan A, et al. Hybrid approach improves success of chronic total occlusion angioplasty. Heart 2016;102(18):1486–93.
16. Wilson WM, Bagnall AJ, Spratt JC. In case of procedure failure: facilitating future success. Interv Cardiol 2013;5(5):521–32.

17. Xenogiannis I, Choi JW, Alaswad K, et al. Outcomes of subintimal plaque modification in chronic total occlusion percutaneous coronary intervention. Catheter Cardiovasc Interv 2019. https://doi.org/10.1002/ccd.28614.

18. Ybarra LF, Dandona S, Daneault B, et al. Drug-coated balloon after subintimal plaque modification in failed coronary chronic total occlusion percutaneous coronary intervention: a novel concept. Catheter Cardiovasc Interv 2019;96(3):609–13.

Intravascular Ultrasound in Chronic Total Occlusion Percutaneous Coronary Intervention
Solving Ambiguity and Improving Durability

Megha Prasad, MD, MS[a], Akiko Maehara, MD[a,b],
Yousif Ahmad, MD, PhD[a], Allen Jeremias, MD[b,c],
Evan Shlofmitz, DO[b,c], Ajay J. Kirtane, MD[a],
Jeffrey W. Moses, MD[a,c], Khady N. Fall, MD[a],
Gary S. Mintz, MD[a], Dimitri Karmpaliotis, MD, PhD[a],
Ziad A. Ali, MD, DPhil[a,b,c],*

KEYWORDS

- Intravascular ultrasound • Chronic total occlusion • Extraplaque • Intraplaque
- Guidewire crossing • Hybrid algorithm

KEY POINTS

- Intravascular ultrasound during percutaneous coronary intervention of a chronic total occlusion may provide additional spatial information that may facilitate guidewire crossing.
- Identification of key information relating to plaque burden, presence of calcification and vessel remodeling can assist the operator in procedural planning and in navigating the hybrid algorithm, reducing lesion ambiguity.
- Identification of guidewire and equipment relative to the true lumen may facilitate guidewire crossing while reducing extraplaque wire tracking.
- Stent placement and expansion may also be optimized with the use of intravascular ultrasound potentially improving durability.
- After recanalization and stenting of a chronic total occlusion, intravascular ultrasound may help identify any complications or suboptimal findings that may not be readily visible on angiography, potentially improving durability.

INTRODUCTION

Chronic total occlusions (CTOs) continue to be a commonly diagnosed lesion on angiography and represent some of the most anatomically complex lesions, often requiring advanced technical expertise to treat percutaneously.[1–4] At experienced centers with highly skilled operators,

[a] Division of Cardiology, Center for Interventional Vascular Therapy, New York Presbyterian Hospital/Columbia University Irving Medical Center, 177 Fort Washington Avenue, New York, NY 10032, USA; [b] Clinical Trials Center, Cardiovascular Research Foundation, 1700 Broadway, New York, NY 10019, USA; [c] St. Francis Hospital, 100 Port Washington Boulevard, Roslyn, NY 11576, USA
* Corresponding author. Columbia University Medical Center, Cardiovascular Research Foundation, 1700 Broadway, 9th Floor, New York, NY 10019.
E-mail address: zaa2112@columbia.edu

Intervent Cardiol Clin 10 (2021) 75–85
https://doi.org/10.1016/j.iccl.2020.09.006

technical success rates are greater than 90%.[2,3,5,6] An inability to pass a guidewire across the occlusion and into the distal true lumen remains the most common mode of failure for CTO–percutaneous coronary intervention (PCI).[5] To achieve higher success rates, advanced approaches iterating within the hybrid algorithm are important. Although many CTOs may be crossed using an antegrade wire escalation approach, other approaches including antegrade dissection reentry (ADR), retrograde dissection and reentry, and reverse controlled antegrade and retrograde tracking (CART) may be required to improve the CTO–PCI success rate.[5] Intravascular ultrasound (IVUS) imaging provides additional visual information that can be critical to facilitating guidewire crossing and further to optimizing durability of CTO–PCI.

Angiography remains the main imaging modality used in treatment of CTOs, but 2-dimensional angiography is a lumenogram that is unable to provide key 3-dimensional structural information that may facilitate safe and efficient guidewire crossing.[7] Moreover, IVUS imaging can provide key information pertaining to plaque burden, vessel remodeling, and calcification that can help with procedural planning. Identification of guidewire position location relative to the lumen is facilitated by the three-dimensional information provided by IVUS imaging, thereby allowing not only more efficient and controlled guidewire crossing, but also limiting extensive extraplaque wire tracking.[7,8]

Once a CTO has been crossed, IVUS imaging has the potential to provide key additional clinical information to help optimize stenting of the lesion, including determination of stent size, expansion and location, and need for additional lesion-modifying procedures such as atherectomy. Last, IVUS imaging at the end of the procedure will help the operator to detect any suboptimal findings or complications that may not be visualized on angiography, including stent malapposition, underexpansion, and distal edge stent dissections that may compromise the durability of the procedure and lead to adverse outcomes.[8–10]

ANTEGRADE APPROACH

Antegrade Wire Escalation

An antegrade approach is often the initial crossing approach when attempting to percutaneously recanalize a CTO. It is also the primary crossing strategy recommended by the CTO hybrid algorithm.[11–14] Controlled and accurate guidewire manipulation is imperative to both improve and standardize CTO–PCI. IVUS

examination may have a key role in providing additional information to help with successful guidewire crossing from the antegrade approach, minimizing the need for retrograde approaches, which not only requires increased technical expertise, but also may be associated with increased complications. When attempting an antegrade approach, IVUS imaging may be especially helpful in several key scenarios one may encounter during attempts at recanalization of a CTO. IVUS imaging can help to confirm the entry point of the CTO, examine the location of the guidewire in the CTO, and facilitate reentry into the intraplaque place should the wire enter the extraplaque space (Fig. 1).[10,11]

When attempting to cross a CTO antegrade, one may encounter difficulty with wire advancement. The operator may wish to avoid extraplaque wire position, for example, owing to the absence of retrograde options, and direct IVUS guidance may be helpful in traversing the lesion while avoiding the extraplaque space.

Short tip IVUS examination may be used to facilitate antegrade wire escalation by advancing the IVUS catheter onto a workhorse wire up to the CTO cap and using a separate parallel microcatheter and appropriately chosen and angled CTO wire to facilitate crossing.[2,10] The wire may be directed under direct IVUS guidance to cross the CTO while visualizing both the intraplaque and extraplaque spaces to avoid extensive extraplaque wire tracking (Fig. 2A).[1,7,15]

The Cap Is Ambiguous

When analyzing 2-dimensional angiography, one may encounter a CTO with a proximal cap that is ambiguous, making crossing significantly more challenging. An ambiguous cap may be difficult to visualize with simple angiography despite multiple angiographic projections. Contralateral angiography may be helpful in elucidating the entry of a CTO; however, if the operator is still unable to visualize the entry point, IVUS imaging can be used to identify the CTO entrance (see Fig. 1).[7,10] The use of IVUS imaging can help to establish key structural information about the cap, including cap location, degree of calcification, and the size of the target vessel. This information can be useful in helping the operator adjust procedural strategy, including choosing a wire, degree of support needed, and the tip shape that may be favorable to cross the lesion.[16]

First and foremost, when attempting to cross a CTO antegrade, especially when the cap may be ambiguous, IVUS imaging should be used to identify and characterize the cap if a side

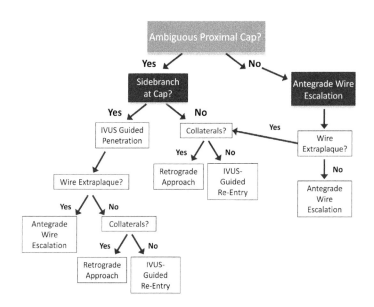

Fig. 1. IVUS for antegrade wire escalation. Stepwise approach using intravascular ultrasound when considering antegrade wire escalation, within the hybrid algorithm, to cross a CTO.

branch is adjacent.[17] This is done by first advancing a workhorse wire into a side branch that is large enough to house an IVUS catheter. The target CTO artery should house a microcatheter and wire near the presumed cap of the CTO. The IVUS catheter can then be advanced to the bifurcation of both arteries on the workhorse wire, and used to identify the CTO cap and visualize the CTO wire.[18] The cap can be assessed for location and calcification to help choose an appropriate wire and wire tip for crossing, ultimately enhancing directionality. With an 8F guide catheter, one may perform live puncture of the cap, advancing the CTO wire into the cap with direct IVUS visualization co-registered with live fluoroscopy (see Fig. 2B). This technique can be used to identify and engage an ambiguous cap, but can also

be applied to ostial lesions when the location of the ostium is difficult to identify on 2-dimensional angiography(see Fig. 1).[10] This technique of live IVUS-guided antegrade puncture of the CTO cap has 2 key limitations. First, to perform live IVUS puncture, it is necessary to at least use an 8F guide catheter to house both the microcatheter and an IVUS catheter. A 7F guide catheter may be used with a 5F IVUS catheter, and a 6F guide catheter may be used if no microcatheter is used for crossing. Second, this technique is highly dependent on the angle of the side branch relative to the main vessel of interest, and on the CTO having favorable imaging (see Figs. 2A and B).[10] Shallower angles allow for better visualization of the cap, but as the angle exceeds 90°, IVUS-guided visualization may not be feasible. In such cases, the operator

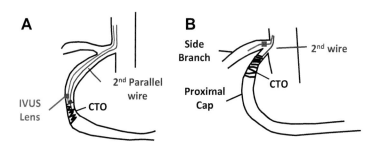

Fig. 2. (A) IVUS-guided antegrade wire escalation. Schematic depicting use of IVUS during antegrade wire escalation. The IVUS catheter (red) is advanced until the IVUS lens is at the proximal cap of the occlusion can. This maneuver is best performed using a short tip IVUS. A second system, ideally a microcatheter and a parallel wire, is then used to attempt crossing the occlusion under live IVUS guidance. (B) Schematic describing use of IVUS to cross an ambiguous cap from an antegrade approach. The IVUS catheter (red) is positioned in the side branch and the IVUS catheter is than advanced and retracted slightly until the cap is identified. This position is marked by dry cine angiogram for co-registration. If the guide size allows, puncture is performed under live IVUS, otherwise the IVUS is withdrawn and the dry cine used for co-registered directionality.

might identify the location of the cap by identifying the location where there is a step-up of the vessel size as the IVUS probe is pulled back from the side branch.[7] Additionally, significant calcification may obscure imaging such that visualization of the proximal cap is not reliable.

ANTEGRADE DISSECTION REENTRY

Many CTOs may be crossed with an antegrade passage of the wire through the true lumen, but when this is not feasible, careful use of the hybrid algorithm can ensure both increased technical success and safety. Most anatomically complex lesions require application of additional technical approaches.[2,12] ADR may provide a safe and efficient way of crossing a CTO lesion, especially if hematoma is minimized and reentry is performed in an optimal location.[13] ADR involves either intentional or accidental wire passage into the extraplaque place, followed by reentry into the true lumen.[19,20] A variety of tools may be used to reenter into the true lumen including specific tapered tip, high penetration force guidewires shaped with an angled tip, a Crossboss catheter (Boston Scientific, Marlborough, MA), a Stingray balloon (Boston Scientific) to facilitate wire reentry, and/or a dual lumen microcatheter.[21] IVUS examination is an additional important modality that should be strongly considered when performing ADR as it can help to directly visualize the directionality of the true lumen, and the most proximal point of transition with favorable characteristics (Fig. 3A). The characteristics include minimal plaque calcification and largest most proximal true lumen area. Dry cineangiography of this position should be performed and marked, without subsequent table movement, to identify the optimal puncture site (see Fig. 3B–D). IVUS examination may be specifically useful in several commonly encountered situations that may require reentry.[10,19,20]

My Antegrade Wire Is Extraplaque
As an antegrade wire is advanced when attempting to cross a CTO via the antegrade approach, the first guidewire may become extraplaque.

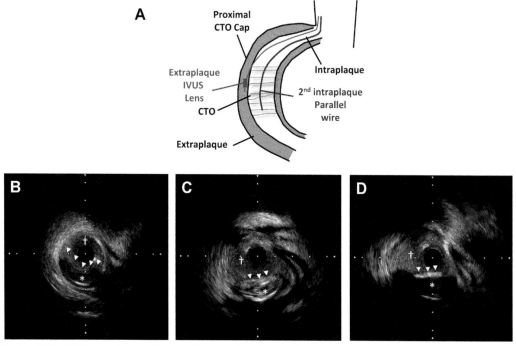

Fig. 3. ADR. (A) Schematic describing ADR under imaging guidance. In the extraplaque space (*pink*), the IVUS catheter (*red*) is loaded on the extraplaque wire. A second intraplaque parallel wire and microcatheter are then used to attempt reentry by directly visualizing both the extraplaque and intraplaque space. (B–D) IVUS may also be used to guide dissection reentry. Extraplaque IVUS identifies the ideal reentry puncture site, showing (B) clear delineation of the medial layer (*arrows*) and true lumen (*asterisk*). IVUS may also identify suboptimal sites such as in (C) heavily diseased (*arrows*) and negatively remodeled site with small true lumen (*asterisk*) and (D) heavily calcified medial layer (*arrows*) with obscuring of the true lumen (*asterisk*). †An intramural hematoma.

This may happen even when attempting to cross a CTO under direct live IVUS visualization or fluoroscopy. Alternatively, when an antegrade approach fails, the operator may opt to knuckle the antegrade guidewire to intentionally advance within the extraplaque space.[21]

In such situations, IVUS visualization may play a key role in not only identifying the location of the wire relative to the intraplaque space, but also in helping to redirect a wire from the extraplaque to the intraplaque space. Especially after extensive wiring attempts, the distal true lumen may be difficult to visualize via retrograde injections, and antegrade injections are to be avoided owing to risk of pressurizing the low resistance extraplaque space and causing extensive hematoma formation.[22] IVUS visualization can thus help to confirm the intraplaque location of the wire before advancing of microcatheters and/or other equipment, reducing risk of dissection propagation and/or unintentional dilation of the extraplaque space.[23]

To redirect an extraplaque wire to the intraplaque space, one should first attempt to advance the IVUS catheter onto the extraplaque wire. If this is not feasible, then a 1.0 mm or 1.5 mm balloon can be used to carefully dilate the extraplaque space to accommodate the IVUS catheter,[24] although this maneuver will contribute to hematoma formation. Ideally, an IVUS catheter with short tip–transducer distance and low crossing profile is used to minimize distal separation of the vessel layers. Once the IVUS catheter is in an appropriate location in the extraplaque plane, a second system with a mirocatheter and second supportive, stiff wire can be advanced into the intraplaque space. The presence of branches and layers including the intima and media can help to confirm that the wire is intraplaque. Similarly, the extraplaque space lacks side-branches and a media and intima layer surrounding the lumen.[18,25] An intramural hematoma may be visualized on IVUS imaging (see Fig. 3B–D). As the IVUS catheter is advanced, the operator must then identify the entry point of the wire entering from the intraplaque space into the extraplaque space and study the relation between the entry point and the relation to any side branches that may be adjacent to the point of the entry.[20,26] Using live fluoroscopy and direct IVUS guidance with the IVUS catheter in the extraplaque space, the second wire can be carefully redirected into the intraplaque space, adjusting the tip and wire as needed based on IVUS imaging (Fig. 4). Reentry under direct IVUS guidance

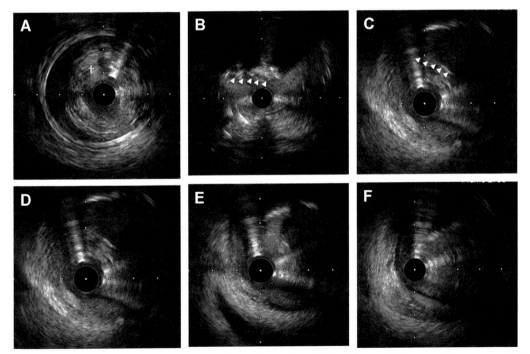

Fig. 4. IVUS images of ADR. Images of ADR performed under live IVUS guidance. (A) Intramural hematoma. (B, C) The intraplaque space (arrows). The extraplaque space is also visualized with several wires. (D–F) The reentry transition.

helps to prevent extensive traversing of the extraplaque space, because this may be associated with worse outcomes.[26–28]

There are some key logistic considerations that should be understood before using IVUS guidance for reentry. First, enlargement of the extraplaque space with the IVUS catheter and an additional balloon at times is a key limitation of this technique, and operators may choose a retrograde approach before dilation of the extraplaque space. Additionally, as described elsewhere in this article, the antegrade guide catheter should be at least 8F to accommodate a microcatheter and an IVUS catheter without significant interaction. With smaller guide catheter sizes, reentry can be performed using a recorded pullback and frequent readvancement of the IVUS catheter to determine location of the wire relative to the true lumen during attempted crossing, or by removing the microcatheter to allow space for the IVUS catheter, although these tactics introduce additional steps of manipulation where position may be lost and compromise efficiency.

RETROGRADE APPROACH

Although an antegrade approach may be an initial crossing strategy used, anatomically complex lesions may require an alternate approach, and thus proficiency in safe and efficient retrograde crossing is important to maximize CTO–PCI success rates.[12] In the event of antegrade failure, opting for a retrograde approach in which the operator has antegrade access to the proximal cap and retrograde access to the distal cap optimizes the chances of successful crossing especially in ambiguous or difficult anatomic subsets.[29] Specifically, CART involves antegrade wiring through the CTO after a retrograde iatrogenic balloon-induced dissection.[6,12,30] The advantage of CART is that it allows limited tracking in the extraplaque place at the site of the CTO lesion and helps with reentry into the distal true lumen.[14] Another approach, reverse CART, involves retrograde dissection past the distal cap using a balloon, and then negotiation of a retrograde support catheter over a dissecting wire near the proximal cap. Antegrade dilation of the extraplaque space is performed using an antegrade balloon with subsequent inflations and ultimate connection of the 2 dissections, allowing retrograde wiring into the proximal true lumen. The success of this technique is dictated by appropriately sized balloon dilation inside the CTO to ensure enough space for reentry.[10,30]

Although these retrograde techniques require additional skill and technical expertise, IVUS visualization has the potential to facilitate use of these advanced approaches to cross a CTO both safely and efficiently.[29] IVUS visualization is especially useful in addressing commonly encountered difficulties with these approaches including situations when the retrograde wire remains in the true lumen, or when the antegrade and retrograde wire are not in the same extraplaque space (see **Fig. 4**).[1] IVUS visualization can be critical in adjusting balloon size, the position of antegrade and retrograde wires, and improving understanding of plaque morphology and wire position to increase the chances of successful crossing.

Antegrade Wire and Retrograde Wire Do Not Connect

When attempting to cross a CTO using a retrograde approach, there may be problems encountered during advancement of the retrograde wire. In addition to reattempting antegrade crossing with additional IVUS guidance, the operator may proceed to attempt true-to-true retrograde crossing or reverse CART to successfully cross the CTO, depending on the anatomy.[31]

To proceed with retrograde crossing, it is important to determine the relative location of the antegrade and retrograde wire. The antegrade and retrograde wire may both be extraplaque, both be intraplaque, or one may be intraplaque and the other may be extraplaque (**Fig. 5**). To visualize this configuration, the IVUS catheter should be advanced into the proximal cap over the antegrade wire, predilating first with a small balloon if needed.[29] Again, for this approach a short-tipped IVUS probe is preferable to better identify the location of the cap and wires. The operator may then use the information regarding wire location relative to the true lumen retrieved by IVUS visualization to understand the spatial relation of both the antegrade and retrograde wires, and the mechanism preventing wire advancement.[32] Identification of plaque characteristics such as heavy calcification may help the operator to revise their strategy as needed. If the retrograde wire is noted to be intraplaque, the operator may continue to attempt true-to-true retrograde crossing, adjusting the wire and the tip as needed. If the wire is extraplaque, the retrograde wire can be redirected to attempt a true to true crossing (**Fig. 6A**).

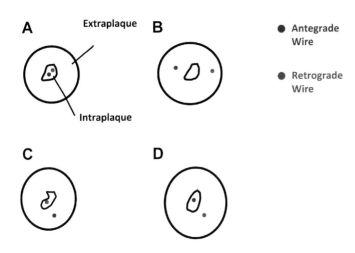

A
Extraplaque

Intraplaque

B

C

D

● Antegrade Wire

● Retrograde Wire

Fig. 5. (A) shows both antegarde and retrograde wires in true lumen. (B) shows that both antegrade and retrograde wires are extraplaque. (C) shows that the retrograde wire is intraplaque and the antegrade wire is extraplaque. (D) shows that the antegrade wire is intraplaque and the retrograde wire is extraplaque.

Retrograde Wire Does Not Advance into the Proximal True Lumen

At times, despite dilation with moderate sized (3.0 mm) antegrade balloons, the retrograde wire may not advance into the proximal true lumen. IVUS visualization can be helpful in ensuring that a correctly size balloon is being used; a common failure mode is an undersized balloon in reverse CART. Moreover, the position of each of the wires is important when performing reverse CART, and IVUS visualization can help to identify the location of the wires relative to the true lumen (see Fig. 5). Reverse CART is simplest when both the antegrade and retrograde wires are in the extraplaque (subintimal) space, and IVUS visualization can help to identify if either wire is in the true lumen, as well as aid in appropriate sizing to larger balloons.[32] Additionally, coronary calcification is associated with failure of reverse CART, and IVUS visualization can be used to choose an appropriate location for reverse CART. Live IVUS guidance may also

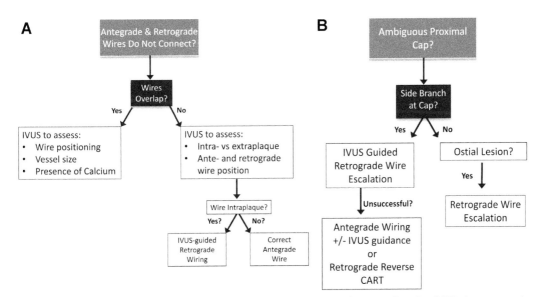

Fig. 6. IVUS for retrograde approach. (A) Flow chart describing key considerations for using IVUS when attempting to cross a CTO from the retrograde approach. IVUS may be helpful when there is difficulty making the antegrade and retrograde wires connect. (B) Flow diagram describing use of IVUS to cross an ambiguous proximal cap and/or ostial lesion via the retrograde approach.

help the operator to advance a retrograde wire to directly puncture the antegrade balloon in an attempt to cross the lesion (see Fig. 6A).

Thus, when true to true retrograde crossing is not feasible owing to difficulty with wire advancement, retrograde dissection and reentry may be necessary to successfully cross the lesion, and IVUS imaging may be helpful during CART and reverse CART as an improved understanding of the size of the vessel may help the operator choose an appropriately sized balloon for reverse CART dilation to successfully connect the 2 wires.[7,25] Additionally, IVUS visualization can help to select an optimal location within the vessel to connect the antegrade and retrograde wires relative to calcification or other vessel characteristics.[32]

There Is an Ambiguous Proximal Cap

An ambiguous proximal cap may pose technical challenges even when crossing a CTO from the retrograde approach.[7,8] It is first important to study the angiogram in detail and determine whether there is a side branch at the cap. If a side branch is present, then IVUS-guided retrograde wire escalation may be performed to ensure that the side branch is avoided (see Fig. 6B). This goal can be accomplished with an antegrade wire and IVUS catheter in the side branch, allowing visualization of the retrograde wire as it is advanced. This maneuver allows the operator to understand the location of the retrograde wire relative to the side branch. If this strategy is unsuccessful, then the operator may consider reattempting antegrade wire escalation using IVUS guidance or may opt to approach the lesion via a retrograde approach.[16]

The Lesion Is Ostial

Another common scenario often encountered by CTO operators is an ostial CTO with no side branch at the cap (see Fig. 6B). These lesions can be technically challenging because an antegrade option is often not favorable owing to limited information from angiography. IVUS visualization plays a key role in facilitating crossing in patients with ostial lesions.[22] A short tip IVUS catheter may be placed in the antegrade cap allowing visualization and characterization of the proximal cap. The retrograde wire can then be advanced under direct IVUS visualization from the proximal cap while avoiding dissection into a main branch. For example, when attempting to cross an ambiguous proximal left anterior descending cap, retrograde wire escalation may result in dissection of the left main artery can be

catastrophic. As such, verification of true lumen passing through the left main is mandatory before completing PCI on the wire achieved via retrograde crossing. Antegrade IVUS visualization can thus protect main branch arteries such as the left main while allowing safe and efficient retrograde crossing.[32]

IVUS visualization may thus be useful when attempting to cross a CTO via the retrograde approach as well. IVUS visualization during retrograde crossing is specifically useful to facilitate advancement of the retrograde wire toward a proximal ambiguous cap, identification of wire location relative to the true lumen, IVUS-guided redirection of the wire and balloon sizing during reverse CART, and when attempting to cross an ostial occlusion to help avoid dissection of a main proximal vessel.

HOW I CAN USE INTRAVASCULAR ULTRASOUND IMAGING AFTER CROSSING?

IVUS visualization is equally if not more useful after successful guidewire crossing to plan stenting strategy. IVUS imaging is helpful for stent sizing, to discriminate between plaque burden and negative remodeling, to evaluate for the need of lesion modification techniques such as atherectomy, and to ensure stent expansion and apposition. Often in patients who have undergone antegrade guidewire crossing or any form of dissection reentry, angiographic visualization with contrast may be avoided to prevent propagation of an iatrogenic dissection. IVUS imaging may be used to help guide not only stent sizing but also stent positioning and expansion until a final angiographic picture is taken. Last, IVUS visualization may be helpful in detecting any complications such as distal edge dissections of the stent that may otherwise be difficult to visualize on angiography.

Several studies have analyzed the potential of benefits of IVUS-guided PCI when compared with angiography-guided PCI and have noted improved outcomes in patients in whom IVUS imaging is used as adjunct imaging during PCI.[33–35] Several large clinical trials and meta-analyses have shown important clinical benefits with the use of IVUS imaging during PCI, with additional studies showing cost-effectiveness of IVUS-guided PCI especially in high-risk patients such as those with CTOs.[28]

Many investigators have previously questioned the durability of CTO–PCI and IVUS imaging has the potential to optimize stent implantation by helping identify appropriate distal landing zone, optimizing stent expansion and minimizing the number of stents required.[7] Furthermore, IVUS visualization may help to detect a distal edge dissection and/or hematoma or other intraprocedural events that may be associated with adverse outcomes. Stent underexpansion has been shown to be a key risk factor in the development of in stent restenosis, and thus stent optimization remains key to optimizing durability of CTO–PCI.[33,36–38] This factor is especially important in patients with CTOs owing to the increased number of stents that may be required, further increasing the risk of stent-related complications including in-stent restenosis. Use of IVUS visualization thus has the potential to improve the operator's ability to detect suboptimal stent results including under expansion and improve long-term durability.[38,39]

WHAT TECHNOLOGY IS ON THE HORIZON?

There are several novel technologies that continue to be developed that may be particularly applicable to CTO–PCI. Incorporation of these advances in technology may help provide additional information to CTO operators in a more efficient and user-friendly fashion. When considering IVUS-guided wiring, there are 2 main limitations in the current practice of CTO operators. First, IVUS visualization does not provide data showing the course of the distal vessel, and multiple angiographic projections are necessary to visualize the entire course of the vessel distal to the occlusion.[10] Also, IVUS visualization is only applicable in the presence of optimal side branches with appropriate anatomy, size, and angle relative to the occlusion. The diameter of the IVUS catheter and the occasional need to dilate the subintimal space continues to be a concern, forcing operators to often consider a retrograde approach before IVUS-guided crossing, and this is largely driven by the fact that the distal end of the current IVUS catheter must reside 2.5 to 23.0 mm distal to the transducer. The need to image from the side limits use of IVUS visualization in CTO–PCI, and dedicated technology with antegrade imaging distal to the catheter tip may help to eliminate need for optimal side branches or excessive subintimal dilation.

Emerging IVUS technology allowing 3-dimensional reconstructions of the vessel allowing distal vessel visualization and displaying real-time road maps of an occluded vessel may help to facilitate crossing. Additionally, potential future use of IVUS catheters with the ability to perform radiofrequency ablation at the catheter tip may have a role in facilitating crossing during simultaneous imaging.

The recent introduction of the CTO-specific IVUS system (AnteOwl IVUS) may further optimize the use of IVUS in CTO–PCI. Okamura and colleagues[40] have reported significant shorter crossing time and number of punctures with the AO-IVUS-based wiring system. This tailored tip detection method may improve a CTO operator's ability to perform IVUS-based 3D wiring to help efficiently and safely cross complex CTOs. Because accurate guidewire control is key to improving efficient and safe guidewire crossing, technology that has the potential to provide increased spatial information regarding guidewire position to the CTO operator using an integrated and user-friendly platform is appealing. The tip detection method developed by Okamura and colleagues addressed several key limitations of previous IVUS technology. The system allows observation of the guidewire tip as well as the shaft of the wire during advancement. The pullback system allows real-time observation and transducer pull back by 15 cm of the guidewire tip as well as the shaft.[40] Additionally, a short tip to transducer length allows more accurate visualization, and the diameter of the tip has been decreased by using a contrast agent in the tip without the marker band. This system also has a reduced diameter that can be used with a 7F guide catheter and a Corsair microcatheter. These improvements have tailored this system for CTO–PCI and IVUS-guided wiring.[40]

Thus, new technology that may improve imaging beyond the catheter tip, visualization of the distal vessel, allow antegrade imaging, and reduce the need for optimal side branches and extensive extraplaque dilation for adequate visualization may have the potential to revolutionize current use of imaging in CTO–PCI and allow it to be more frequently adopted during interventions that may be optimized by additional imaging.[10,32,40]

SUMMARY

IVUS visualization thus has the potential to facilitate guidewire crossing as an operator navigates the hybrid algorithm during CTO–PCI, and may help to optimize success rates by providing additional spatial information that are especially useful in certain scenarios, including the presence of an ostial lesion or ambiguous cap, or to help understand options to proceed when the antegrade wire is extraplaque or when both antegrade and retrograde wires are in different planes. It also has the potential to improve durability by providing additional information regarding stent placement and expansion. Novel technology addressing current limitations has the potential to further improve utility of IVUS visualization in CTO–PCI.

CLINICAL CARE POINTS

- Complex coronary operators should be familiar with intravascular ultrasound and use it to improve success rates of CTO-PCI.
- Intravascular ultrasound may be used for procedural planning, guidewire crossing, stent deployment and optimization and detection of suboptimal results including distal edge dissection or thrombus.
- Detection of extraplaque wire position by intravascular ultrasound is important to limit subintimal tracking and faciliate re-entry.
- A larger guide should be used to accomodate both a microcatheter with a wire and an imaging catheter for direct ultrasound-guided puncture.
- Familiarity with intravascular ultrasound imaging including detection of wire position, understanding of lesion morphology and vessel sizing can play a key role in improving success and durability of CTO-PCI.

REFERENCES

1. Dai J, Katoh O, Kyo E, et al. Approach for chronic total occlusion with intravascular ultrasound-guided reverse controlled antegrade and retrograde tracking technique: single center experience. J Interv Cardiol 2013;26(5):434–43.
2. Namazi MH, Serati AR, Vakili H, et al. A novel risk score in predicting failure or success for antegrade approach to percutaneous coronary intervention of chronic total occlusion: antegrade CTO score. Int J Angiol 2017;26(2):89–94.
3. Su YM, Pan M, Geng HH, et al. Outcomes after percutaneous coronary intervention and comparison among scoring systems in predicting procedural success in elderly patients (≥75 years) with chronic total occlusion. Coron Artery Dis 2019; 30(7):481–7.
4. Tan KH, Sulke N, Taub NA, et al. Determinants of success of coronary angioplasty in patients with a chronic total occlusion: a multiple logistic

regression model to improve selection of patients. Br Heart J 1993;70(2):126–31.
5. Cummings DM, Letter AJ, Howard G, et al. Medication adherence and stroke/TIA risk in treated hypertensives: results from the REGARDS study. J Am Soc Hypertens 2013;7(5):363–9.
6. Wilson WM, Walsh SJ, Yan AT, et al. Hybrid approach improves success of chronic total occlusion angioplasty. Heart 2016;102(18):1486–93.
7. Galassi AR, Sumitsuji S, Boukhris M, et al. Utility of intravascular ultrasound in percutaneous revascularization of chronic total occlusions: an overview. JACC Cardiovasc Interv 2016;9(19):1979–91.
8. Mashayekhi K, Behnes M. The role of intravascular ultrasound in the treatment of chronic total occlusion with percutaneous coronary intervention. Cardiol J 2020;27(1):4–5.
9. Zhang Y, Farooq V, Garcia-Garcia HM, et al. Comparison of intravascular ultrasound versus angiography-guided drug-eluting stent implantation: a meta-analysis of one randomised trial and ten observational studies involving 19,619 patients. EuroIntervention 2012;8(7):855–65.
10. Dash D, Li L. Intravascular ultrasound guided percutaneous coronary intervention for chronic total occlusion. Curr Cardiol Rev 2015;11(4). 323-317.
11. Basir MB, Karatasakis A, Alqarqaz M, et al. Further validation of the hybrid algorithm for CTO PCI; difficult lesions, same success. Cardiovasc Revasc Med 2017;18(5):328–31.
12. McNeice A, Ladwiniec A, Walsh S, et al. Hybrid approach to percutaneous coronary intervention to treat chronic total occlusions. Eur Cardiol 2017; 12(1):46–51.
13. Rangan BV, Kotsia A, Christopoulos G, et al. The hybrid approach for intervention of chronic total occlusions. Curr Cardiol Rev 2015;11(4):299–304.
14. Tajti P, Brilakis ES. Does the hybrid algorithm has real impact on long-term outcomes or should only be used as a valuable approach for CTO crossing? J Thorac Dis 2018;10(3):1320–4.
15. Matsubara T, Murata A, Kanyama H, et al. IVUS-guided wiring technique: promising approach for the chronic total occlusion. Catheter Cardiovasc Interv 2004;61(3):381–6.
16. Park Y, Park HS, Jang GL, et al. Intravascular ultrasound guided recanalization of stumpless chronic total occlusion. Int J Cardiol 2011;148(2):174–8.
17. Fujii K, Ochiai M, Mintz GS, et al. Procedural implications of intravascular ultrasound morphologic features of chronic total coronary occlusions. Am J Cardiol 2006;97(10):1455–62.
18. Furuichi S, Airoldi F, Colombo A. Intravascular ultrasound-guided wiring for chronic total occlusion. Catheter Cardiovasc Interv 2007;70(6):856–9.
19. Maeremans J, Dens J, Spratt JC, et al. Antegrade dissection and reentry as part of the hybrid chronic

total occlusion revascularization strategy: a sub-analysis of the RECHARGE Registry (Registry of CrossBoss and Hybrid Procedures in France, the Netherlands, Belgium and United Kingdom). Circ Cardiovasc Interv 2017;10(6):e004791.

20. Wyman RM. Antegrade dissection and reentry: tools and techniques. Interv Cardiol Clin 2012;1(3): 315–24.

21. Wu EB, Brilakis ES, Lo S, et al. Advances in cross-boss/stingray use in antegrade dissection reentry from the Asia Pacific Chronic Total Occlusion Club. Catheter Cardiovasc Interv 2019. https://doi.org/10.1002/ccd.28607.

22. Wallace EL, Ziada KM. Intravascular-ultrasound assisted localization and revascularization of an ostial chronic total occlusion: utility of near-field and far-field imaging. J Invasive Cardiol 2015; 27(3):E37–9.

23. Chou RH, Lai CH, Lu TM. Side-branch and coaxial intravascular ultrasound guided wire re-entry after failed retrograde approach of chronic total occlusion intervention. Acta Cardiol Sin 2016;32(3):363–6.

24. Azzalini L, Carlino M, Colombo A. Clinical signifi-cance of intravascular ultrasound-detected vascular injury following chronic total occlusion recanaliza-tion with intraplaque versus subintimal tracking techniques. JACC Cardiovasc Interv 2017;10(15): 1600–1.

25. Huang WC, Teng HI, Hsueh CH, et al. Intravascular ultrasound guided wiring re-entry technique for complex chronic total occlusions. J Interv Cardiol 2018;31(5):572–9.

26. Banerjee S, Master R, Brilakis ES. Intravascular ultrasound-guided true lumen re-entry for success-ful recanalization of chronic total occlusions. J Invasive Cardiol 2010;22(12):608–10.

27. Finn MT, Doshi D, Cleman J, et al. Intravascular ultrasound analysis of intraplaque versus subinti-mal tracking in percutaneous intervention for cor-onary chronic total occlusions: one year outcomes. Catheter Cardiovasc Interv 2019;93(6): 1048–56.

28. Song L, Maehara A, Finn MT, et al. Intravascular ul-trasound analysis of intraplaque versus subintimal tracking in percutaneous intervention for coronary chronic total occlusions and association with proce-dural outcomes. JACC Cardiovasc Interv 2017; 10(10):1011–21.

29. Tsujita K, Maehara A, Mintz GS, et al. Intravascular ultrasound comparison of the retrograde versus antegrade approach to percutaneous intervention for chronic total coronary occlusions. JACC Cardio-vasc Interv 2009;2(9):846–54.

30. DeMartini TJ. Retrograde dissection reentry for coronary chronic total occlusions. Interv Cardiol Clin 2012;1(3):339–44.

31. Ying LH, Fan YS, Lu Y, et al. Intravascular ultrasound guided retrograde guidewire true lumen tracking technique for chronic total occlusion intervention. J Geriatr Cardiol 2018;15(2):199–202.

32. Rathore S, Katoh O, Tuschikane E, et al. A novel modification of the retrograde approach for the recanalization of chronic total occlusion of the cor-onary arteries intravascular ultrasound-guided reverse controlled antegrade and retrograde tracking. JACC Cardiovasc Interv 2010;3(2): 155–64.

33. Jensen LO, Vikman S, Antonsen L, et al. Intravas-cular ultrasound assessment of minimum lumen area and intimal hyperplasia in in-stent restenosis after drug-eluting or bare-metal stent implantation. The Nordic Intravascular Ultrasound Study (NIVUS). Cardiovasc Revasc Med 2017;18(8):577–82.

34. Hong MK, Lee CW, Kim JH, et al. Impact of various intravascular ultrasound criteria for stent optimiza-tion on the six-month angiographic restenosis. Catheter Cardiovasc Interv 2002;56(2):178–83.

35. Yoon HJ, Hur SH. Optimization of stent deploy-ment by intravascular ultrasound. Korean J Intern Med 2012;27(1):30–8.

36. Yin D, Mintz GS, Song L, et al. In-stent restenosis characteristics and repeat stenting underexpan-sion: insights from optical coherence tomography. EuroIntervention 2020;16(4):e335–43.

37. Sakamoto T, Kawarabayashi T, Taguchi H, et al. Intravascular ultrasound-guided balloon angio-plasty for treatment of in-stent restenosis. Catheter Cardiovasc Interv 1999;47(3):298–303.

38. Funada R, Oikawa Y, Yajima J, et al. Prediction of late restenosis after sirolimus-eluting stent implan-tation using serial quantitative angiographic and intravascular ultrasound analysis. Cardiovasc Interv Ther 2011;26(1):26–32.

39. Moussa I, Moses J, Di Mario C, et al. Does the spe-cific intravascular ultrasound criterion used to opti-mize stent expansion have an impact on the probability of stent restenosis? Am J Cardiol 1999;83(7):1012–7.

40. Okamura A, Iwakura K, Iwamoto M, et al. Tip detec-tion method using the new IVUS facilitates the 3-Dimensional wiring technique for CTO interven-tion. JACC Cardiovasc Interv 2020;13(1):74–82.

The Hybrid Approach and Its Variations for Chronic Total Occlusion Percutaneous Coronary Intervention

Craig A. Thompson, MD, MMSc[a,b,c,d,*]

KEYWORDS

- Hybrid approach • Chronic total occlusion • Percutaneous coronary intervention

KEY POINTS

- Selected patients with coronary chronic total occlusion (CTO) benefit with respect to symptoms, quality of life, ischemia reduction, and potentially longevity among other benefits.
- CTO lesions tend to be the most technically challenging for practicing interventional cardiologists to deliver a successful and safe result and clinical experience for a given patient.
- The Hybrid algorithm for CTO percutaneous coronary intervention and the subsequent subalgorithms for focused technical challenges have a standardized process and provide a consistent platform for optimized patient care, medical education, and clinical investigation in patients challenged with total occlusion and complex coronary disease.

INTRODUCTION

Percutaneous coronary intervention (PCI) of chronic total occlusions (CTO) has long been a challenge and often a limiter for optimal coronary revascularization. These challenges historically are multifactorial but include technical complexity, periodically differential procedural risks, educational paradigms, and misunderstanding of the value of successful CTO PCI procedures in well-selected patients by the clinical community. The variability in care a given patient receives can be vastly different depending on the access to accomplished and prepared CTO PCI programs. Often the patients receive stand-alone medical therapy or are referred for coronary artery bypass surgery, when PCI could be a superior option for many. The development of the first standardized algorithm, the hybrid algorithm for CTO PCI,[1–3] provided a much-needed platform to technically approach complex patients with CTO, which serves to minimize variability, enhance technical outcomes, improve safety, and facilitate research and education. As adoption has grown, variants of an algorithmic approach have surfaced in many geographies across the globe to meet the regional needs, technology access, and sensibilities.

DEVELOPMENT OF THE HYBRID ALGORITHM FOR CHRONIC TOTAL OCCLUSION PERCUTANEOUS CORONARY INTERVENTION

The hybrid algorithm was largely conceived circa 2008 to 2010 and ultimately codified at the "Bellingham Summit" with a group of CTO expert operators in January 2011. Five operators double scrubbed cases with the other physicians supporting as panelists. The objective was to distill simple findings from the angiogram and

[a] Interventional Cardiology, NYU Langone Health System, New York City, NY, USA; [b] Cardiac Catheterization Laboratories, NYU Langone Health System, New York City, NY, USA; [c] Cardiac Catheterization Laboratories, NYU Langone-Tisch Hospital, New York City, NY, USA; [d] New York University School of Medicine, New York City, NY, USA
* 550 1st Avenue, 14th Floor, New York, NY 10016.
E-mail address: Craig.Thompson@nyulangone.org

Intervent Cardiol Clin 10 (2021) 87–91
https://doi.org/10.1016/j.iccl.2020.09.013

use these to guide a tailored, sequential approach of primary, secondary, and tertiary strategies that could, and were, defined before the procedure. Over the course of 3 days, this method was successful in 17/17 patients across the 5 operators with disparate backgrounds. Ultimately, the commonality and consistency of messaging promoted better educational, developmental, and investigational in addition to outstanding outcomes. In a relatively short timeframe, additional series of patients such as the Hybrid Live case registry,[4] with more than 150 live recorded adjudicated procedures, and other studies like the OPEN CTO registry[5–8] continued to provide valuable information, particularly with the consistency and ability to somewhat neutralize the effects of more complex disease on technical success.

THE FOUR FUNDAMENTAL QUESTIONS

Four questions are asked of the initial diagnostic and/or multiple simultaneous catheter injections of the coronary anatomy to define initial and subsequent procedural approaches:

1. Ambiguity of the proximal cap (can one clarify with certainty with angiography or intravascular ultrasound the proximal cap of the CTO?)
2. Lesion length (<> 20 mm; longer lesions less often successful or efficient with wire strategies alone)
3. Distal target (is the distal vessel reasonably healthy enough to wire or reenter as needed?)
4. Interventional collaterals (are there collaterals that are safe and reasonable within a given operators experience and skillset?)

The objective of the 4 questions is to identify the key technical parameters that will best match and balance safety, success, and efficient workflow. There are many patients in whom several technical methods could likely be successful and a nontrivial minority whereby options become progressively limited. This reason is key to having a broad "toolkit" and skillsets. *The decision, in an expert CTO operator's hands, to proceed with CTO PCI should be linked to patient-based need, not the angiogram!* In an ideal setting, the patient need determines whether we move forward with PCI…the angiogram merely provides for technical details of how to best accomplish the goal.

The 4 aforementioned lesion characteristics are identified, balanced, and distilled into the algorithm process (**Fig. 1**), which creates a success-safety hierarchy with initial planned and provisional strategies. Fundamentally, there are 4 CTO revascularization strategies/methods: antegrade wire escalation (AWE), antegrade dissection reentry (ADR), retrograde wire escalation (RWE), and retrograde dissection reentry (RDR).

The wire escalation (AWE, RWE) strategies are typically the starting options for relatively short (<20 mm) lesions, and AWE itself, even in the current era, comprises most cases in most practices. A typical lesion for AWE, for instance, is a useful initial strategy in short lesions with no ambiguity at the proximal cap and a reasonable distal target. The wires are classified according to the use case, of which there are three: (1) a probing soft wire to explore the CTO; (2) a moderate tip weight polymer jacketed wire (examples, Pilot 200 [Abbott Vascular] Gladius and Gladius Mongo [Asahi Intecc]) for long lesions and dissections; (3) penetration wires for CTO access and to cross short distances when the vessel course is clear (Hornet 14, Boston Scientific, Maple Grove, MN, USA; Confianza Pro 12g [Asahi Intecc]).

Dissection reentry strategies, for all intents and purposes, are use of the Stingray reentry system (Boston Scientific), or occasionally, Subintimal Tracking and Reentry (STAR) in the antegrade direction, and Reverse Controlled Antegrade Retrograde Tracking (Reverse CART), or CART in the retrograde direction. These methods can overcome anatomic complexity and technical challenges.

The CrossBoss support catheter, and the Stingray Balloon catheter and wire system, is a dedicated CTO crossing and reentry system for ADR (https://www.bostonscientific.com/en-US/products/cto-systems/stingray-cto-balloon-catheter-and-guidewire.html) and can be used in isolation or together. The crux of the reentry portion, the stingray balloon, is a 1-mm flat balloon that is placed in the subadventitial or intraplaque space with exit ports 180° apart to facilitate reentry to the distal true lumen.[9,10] The STAR technique can be useful for bailout when other methods fail, to rescue side branches, and to allow for vessel preparation (Subintimal Plaque Modification) for failing procedures with planned second-stage follow-up attempt. The STAR method involves a polymer jacketed wire that is looped ("knuckled") and advanced within the vessel architecture with the goal of distal reentry when the path of least resistance allows the wire to reenter the true lumen. Although initially this method was plagued with durability concerns, better patient

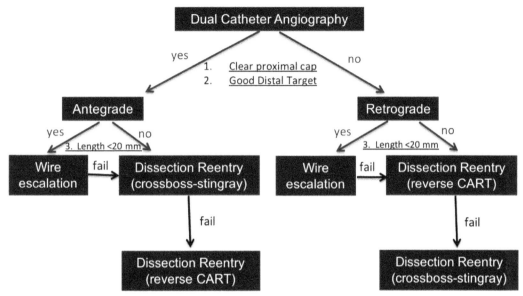

Fig. 1. Initial and provisional approaches for hybrid CTO PCI. (*Courtesy of* Craig Thompson.)

and lesion selection, attention to multivessel outflow, and newer technologies (eg, Gladius Mongo, Asahi Intecc) have allowed this technique to find a valuable clinical home in very well-selected, refractory cases.

For RDR, the most common method is reverse CART. With this approach, a retrograde catheter is approximated to an antegrade balloon system, with the intent to connect the channels. Once crossed, an externalized wire provides full control of the subtended vascular bed. There are variants of reverse CART, but this is most common (**Fig. 2**). On occasion, the balloon can be placed retrograde with an attempt to wire from the antegrade direction ("classic CART"), which can be useful. In addition, a combination of approaches "Facilitated ADR" can be performed using advantages of both antegrade and retrograde methods in selected complex situations.

Although the step-by-step technical details of these 4 methods are beyond the scope of this article, they are well described in the peer-reviewed medical literature and represented in many CTO specialty conferences.

The major principles of the Hybrid Algorithm for CTO PCI are as follows:

1. The algorithm provides a consistent "playbook" of what to do when, for an operator and team that are comfortable with the requisite underlying skillsets (ADR/AWE/RDR/RWE).
2. It exploits conditional probability that incorporates the most likely safe, successful, and efficient initial and provisional approaches.
3. It switches rapidly within a given technique or between techniques to optimize success, safety, and efficiency.
4. It considers equipoise in long-term outcomes between the underlying techniques when adjusted for disease burden and clinical comorbidities.

The underlying techniques, supportive technologies, and data in the intervening years continue to develop. Since the inception of Hybrid CTO PCI, additional treatment pathways, "the Algorithms of the Algorithm," have been developed to standardize challenges that operators encounter in CTO and Complex PCI procedures.[11] These learnings, largely developed and standardized within the CTO community, have broad applicability across broad swaths of complex coronary disease and PCI. *It is incredibly important to maintain a patient-centric approach and to realize that CTO PCI is an extension of complex coronary disease, and the goal is to achieve an optimized technical*

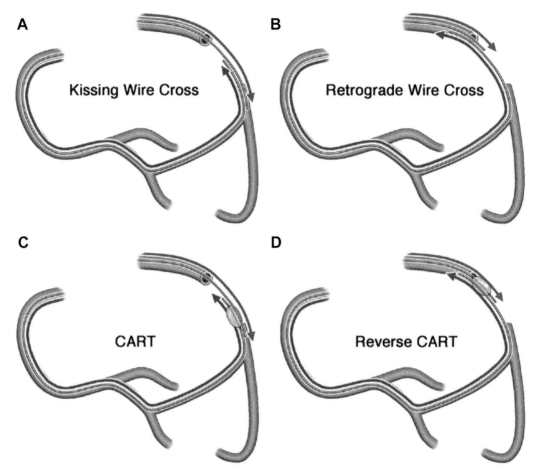

Fig. 2. Methods for CTO crossing using the retrograde approach. (*From* Satoru Sumitsuji, Katsumi Inoue, Masahiko Ochiai, et al. Fundamental Wire Technique and Current Standard Strategy of Percutaneous Intervention for Chronic Total Occlusion with Histopathological Insights JACC: Cardiovascular Interventions, Volume 4, Issue 9, September 2011; with permission.)

outcome that will translate to optimized clinical outcomes.

SUMMARY

Selected patients with coronary CTO benefit with respect to symptoms, quality of life, ischemia reduction, and potential longevity among other benefits. CTO lesions tend to be the most technically challenging for practicing interventional cardiologists to deliver a successful and safe result and clinical experience for a given patient. The Hybrid algorithm for CTO PCI and the subsequent subalgorithms for focused technical challenges have a standardized process and provide a consistent platform for optimized patient care, medical education, and clinical investigation in patients challenged with total occlusion and complex coronary disease.

CLINICS CARE POINTS

- Use of the Hybrid technique has improved success rate of CTO PCI to approximately 90%.
- Reverse CART is the most common method for retrograde CTO PCI techniques, used to solve proximal cap ambiguity and solve long lesions.
- Contemporary ADR has expanded its applications.
- Antegrade wire escalation is limited in regaining reentry to the true lumen in many cases.

- Rapidly changing strategy as challenges are encountered and solved is a key component to success.

REFERENCES

1. Thompson CA. The hybrid approach for percutaneous revascularization of coronary chronic total occlusions. Interv Cardiol Clin 2012;1(3):349–53.
2. Ramanath VS, Thompson CA. Coronary chronic total occlusion recanalisation - current techniques and approaches. Interv Cardiol 2013;8(1):41–5.
3. Thompson CA. Percutaneous revascularization of coronary chronic total occlusions: the new era begins. JACC Cardiovasc Interv 2010;3(2):152–4.
4. Daniels DV, Banerjee S, Alaswad K, et al. Safety and efficacy of the hybrid approach in coronary chronic total occlusion percutaneous coronary intervention: the Hybrid Video Registry. Catheter Cardiovasc Interv 2018;91(2):175–9.
5. Jones DA, Weerackody R, Rathod K, et al. Successful recanalization of chronic total occlusions is associated with improved long-term survival. JACC Cardiovasc Interv 2012;5(4):380–8.
6. Sapontis J, Salisbury AC, Yeh RW, et al. Early procedural and health status outcomes after chronic total occlusion angioplasty: a report from the OPEN-CTO Registry (Outcomes, Patient Health Status, and Efficiency in Chronic Total Occlusion Hybrid Procedures). JACC Cardiovasc Interv 2017; 10(15):1523–34.
7. Khariton Y, Airhart S, Salisbury AC, et al. Health status benefits of successful chronic total occlusion revascularization across the spectrum of left ventricular function: insights from the OPEN-CTO Registry. JACC Cardiovasc Interv 2018;11(22):2276–83.
8. Salisbury AC, Karmpaliotis D, Grantham JA, et al. In-hospital costs and costs of complications of chronic total occlusion angioplasty: insights from the OPEN-CTO Registry. JACC Cardiovasc Interv 2019;12(4):323–31.
9. Whitlow PL, Lombardi WL, Araya M, et al. Initial experience with a dedicated coronary re-entry device for revascularization of chronic total occlusions. Catheter Cardiovasc Interv 2012;80(5): 807–13.
10. Whitlow PL, Burke MN, Lombardi WL, et al. FAST-CTOs Trial Investigators. Use of a novel crossing and re-entry system in coronary chronic total occlusions that have failed standard crossing techniques: results of the FAST-CTOs (Facilitated Antegrade Steering Technique in Chronic Total Occlusions) trial. JACC Cardiovasc Interv 2012;5(4):393–401.
11. Riley RF, Walsh SJ, Kirtane AJ, et al. Algorithmic solutions to common problems encountered during chronic total occlusion angioplasty: the algorithms within the algorithm. Catheter Cardiovasc Interv 2019;93(2):286–97.

Perforation Mechanisms, Risk Stratification, and Management in the Non-post Coronary Artery Bypass Graft Patient

Jennifer A. Tremmel, MD, MS

KEYWORDS

- Coronary occlusion • Coronary perforation • Percutaneous coronary intervention
- Coronary complication • Covered stents • Coils

KEY POINTS

- Perforation occurs in approximately 9% of percutaneous coronary interventions for chronic total occlusions; approximately one-half of these perforations require treatment.
- The diagnosis and management of a coronary perforation is not just based on the visual appearance, but also on an assessment of the hemodynamics.
- A large vessel perforation is generally managed with a covered stent, whereas a distal vessel perforation is generally managed with embolization.

Coronary perforation is a relatively common and potentially lethal complication of percutaneous coronary intervention for chronic total occlusion. One-half of all perforations require treatment, and there are certain features that can signify a more high-risk perforation. If a perforation occurs, the first step is to inflate a balloon to stop the bleeding. In large vessels, this generally involves a covered stent; for smaller vessels, this usually involves embolization. Because there are certain mechanisms known to increase the risk of perforation, steps to minimize these occurrences in the fist place are best.

Coronary perforation is a relatively common and potentially life-threatening complication of chronic total occlusion (CTO) percutaneous coronary intervention (PCI). In fact, CTO PCI is the strongest independent predictor of developing a coronary perforation, with a 7-fold increase in the adjusted risk compared with non-CTO PCI.[1] Among experienced operators in the current era, the incidence of coronary perforation during CTO PCI is approximately 4% to 9%,[2–4] with higher rates occurring in more complex cases and among more specialized CTO operators.[5,6] Patients with a perforation have a significantly higher major adverse cardiac event rate (25.9% vs 1.6%; $P<.001$).[3] Adverse events associated with a perforation include major bleeding, the need for a blood transfusion, myocardial infarction, emergency surgery, and death.[2,3,5] The mortality rate associated with a perforation during CTO PCI is approximately 5% to 10%,[2,4] and even higher among patients with tamponade requiring pericardiocentesis (16.7%).[3] Although only about one-half of perforations during CTO PCI require treatment, for those requiring treatment, the in-hospital mortality rate is nearly 21%.[4]

In addition to the early mortality rate, it has been suggested that perforations during CTO PCI can have a "legacy effect," with a continued excess mortality rate at 12 months and 60 months after the procedure among

Stanford University Medical Center, 300 Pasteur Drive, Room H2103, Stanford, CA 94305, USA
E-mail address: jtremmel@stanford.edu

Intervent Cardiol Clin 10 (2021) 93–99
https://doi.org/10.1016/j.iccl.2020.09.005
2211-7458/21/© 2020 Elsevier Inc. All rights reserved.

perforation survivors compared with matched subjects without a perforation.[5] This legacy effect may be due to several factors, including incomplete revascularization owing to procedure interruption, concomitant complications, and/or restenosis or thrombosis of covered stents, among others. Indeed, having a coronary perforation during CTO PCI is associated with lower technical and procedural success rates, and the target vessel failure rate is markedly higher at 30 days among patients who have suffered a perforation (9.4% vs 1.0%; P<.001).[2,3]

Patient-related risk factors for coronary perforation during CTO PCI include older age, female sex, a history of PCI, and prior coronary artery bypass grafting.[2,3,5] Perforation in patients after coronary artery bypass grafting is discussed in the next article. There is also evidence that the more complex the CTO (a higher J-CTO score, higher PROGRESS-CTO Complications score), the higher the risk of perforation.[2,3] Use of specialized equipment, such as microcatheters, atherectomy, and Crossboss/Stingray may increase the risk of perforation, but this increased risk more likely reflects the complexity of the CTO rather than an inherent danger of the device itself.[3,5] Perforations are more commonly cited as being associated with antegrade dissection reentry and the retrograde approach, although the data regarding the risk of perforation during the retrograde approach may be skewed owing to some studies implicating the retrograde approach simply if it was used during a case, even if it was not the approach resulting in the perforation.[2–4] In addition, as with specialized equipment, the increased risk of perforation with certain approaches may be more about the complexity of the CTO than the strategy itself.

MECHANISMS OF CORONARY PERFORATION

Coronary perforation can occur at any stage of CTO PCI, from initial wiring to post-dilation, and in any segment of the coronary tree (large vessels, distal vessels, septal collaterals, and epicardial collaterals). Perforations in a large vessel are generally due to overdilation, dilation in a calcified vessel, atherectomy, balloon rupture, or equipment exiting the vessel, either over a wire (such as a microcatheter when wire position is not confirmed to be within the vessel architecture) or without a wire (such as a Cross-Boss diverting into a small side branch during advancement). When they occur in a distal vessel, perforations are usually due to a wire exiting the vessel, particularly polymer jacketed

and/or hydrophilic wires, although mechanisms listed for large vessels can also occur in small vessels, and vice versa. In a detailed analysis of perforation mechanisms, 32% of perforations were caused by wire exit (2% at the CTO site, 6% in the distal vessel, and 23% in the retrograde channel) and 29% were caused by microcatheter advancement (7% antegrade and 22% retrograde).[2] Balloon- and stent-induced perforations were observed in 22% and 9% of cases, respectively. Less common were perforations owing to the CrossBoss and rotational atherectomy, although the relative use of these devices in this study was low.

The mechanism of perforation may be related to the strategy being used when the perforation occurred. As mentioned elsewhere in this article, antegrade dissection reentry and a retrograde approach have been associated with a higher rate of perforation but in fact more perforations occur during an antegrade rather than retrograde approach. In the Outcomes, Patient health status, and Efficiency iN Chronic Total Occlusion hybrid procedures (OPEN-CTO) registry, using a detailed core laboratory analysis of patients with an angiographic perforation, 55% of the perforations occurred during the antegrade strategy and 45% occurred during the retrograde strategy.[4] Among the antegrade perforations, 20% occurred during an antegrade wire escalation attempt, whereas 35% occurred during antegrade dissection reentry. Among the retrograde perforations, 21% occurred during a retrograde wire escalation attempt, while 24% occurred during a retrograde dissection reentry attempt. In those patients who had both antegrade and retrograde approaches during their CTO PCI, perforation occurred more commonly (60.1%) during the antegrade attempt. Among the antegrade perforations, major complications occurred more often in more proximal perforations, especially in the right coronary artery, while the frequency of a perforation requiring treatment was lower with distal perforations.

Perforation in the epicardial collaterals appears to be most dangerous. In the OPEN-CTO registry, all perforations that occurred in the epicardial vessels required treatment and one-half resulted in in-hospital death.[4] A single-center study analysis of retrograde PCI via the epicardial collaterals (n = 155) noted a perforation rate of 15.5%.[7] The perforation site was in the CTO target vessel in 29.2% and in the epicardial collateral in 70.8%. Independent predictors of perforation included renal dysfunction, right coronary artery CTO, and an epicardial CTO score of 2 or higher. Tamponade occurred in 29%. At the 7-year follow-up, there was no statistically significant difference in major adverse cardiac event rates between those with versus those without a perforation (16.7% vs 9.9%; P = .484), but instead, success of the CTO PCI was independently associated with fewer major adverse cardiac events.

RISK STRATIFICATION

There are a number of ways of classifying coronary CTO perforations. A traditional risk-based classification schema for perforations was described by Ellis and colleagues[8] in 1994 in response to increased perforations seen with new devices, such as atherectomy and laser. It was based on angiographic appearance, with type I being an extraluminal crater without extravasation, type II being pericardial or myocardial blush without contrast jet extravasation, type III being frank streaming of contrast through an exit hole larger than 1 mm, and cavity spilling being a type III perforation in which the contrast jet extravasation goes into an anatomic cavity (eg, cardiac chamber or coronary sinus). The authors showed that the clinical risk increased with a higher classification, but noted that even low-risk perforations could occasionally have poor outcomes and that patients should be observed for delayed cardiac tamponade for at least 24 hours.

Although the Ellis classification was not developed for CTO PCI, it still has applicability. A retrospective analysis of coronary perforations in 1811 consecutive patients undergoing CTO PCI at 5 European centers between 2011 and 2018 demonstrated that the frequency of Ellis type I, II, III, and III "cavity spilling" perforations was 11%, 46%, 28%, and 14%, respectively.[2] Ellis type III perforations were most likely to require treatment followed by Ellis type II, and then Ellis type I. Ellis type III perforations were also most frequently observed at the CTO site and were accountable for 80% of the tamponades and 60% of the deaths. Septal perforations were benign, regardless of their severity as assessed by the Ellis classification. However, it should be noted that there are case reports of severe complications from septal perforations and no perforation should be taken lightly.[9–11]

Similarly, a retrospective analysis of consecutive patients (n = 2409) from the large multicenter Prospective Global Registry for the Study of Chronic Total Occlusion Intervention (PROGRESS-CTO) registry reported a frequency of Ellis type I, II, and III perforations as 21%, 26%, and 52%, respectively.[3] All Ellis type III

perforations required treatment, whereas 20% of Ellis type II and 37% of Ellis type I did not. The most aggressive treatment with Ellis type I perforations was a prolonged balloon inflation and/or anticoagulation reversal, whereas covered stents, coil embolization, pericardiocentesis, and emergency surgery were commonly needed with Ellis type III perforations, and the in-hospital mortality rate with these more severe perforations was 18%.

A more contemporary schema of perforations specifically for CTO PCI has been developed from an analysis of the OPEN-CTO registry. Each perforation was evaluated by an angiographic core laboratory for maximal area, length, location, shape, presence of staining, speed of filling, speed of drainage, and strategy that caused the perforation. The shape was categorized into 7 patterns (oval, round, spotty, cloud-like, floating, mushroom-like, and around the vessel). Perforations requiring treatment tended to be larger, were more likely in collateral vessels, had a high-risk shape (cloud-like and floating), and were less likely to have staining (fast filling, fast draining). All perforations in epicardial collaterals required treatment. Perforations that were associated with a major adverse event were larger in size, more proximal (most commonly in the right coronary artery) or in a collateral vessel, and had a high-risk shape. In contrast, perforations with less staining, fast filling, and fast draining were not significantly associated with adverse outcomes, suggesting that CTO operators should not be reassured on the basis of the presence of staining and a slow speed of filling and draining alone when encountering coronary perforation, and should give more consideration to location, shape, and size.

Although these risk classifications are angiographic, it should be noted that perforation is not simply a visual diagnosis. One should always be attending to the hemodynamics, which may detect a perforation before it is noted angiographically, particularly because contrast injections are often limited during CTO PCI. If the blood pressure drops, a perforation should be suspected and ruled out. The hemodynamics can also guide one with regard to the need for treatment, or for escalating treatment. Some advocate the placement of a pulmonary artery catheter for closer monitoring. If a perforation seems to be severe angiographically, but the hemodynamics are stable, there may be time to do further diagnostic testing, such as getting an echocardiogram to see if the perforation is contained in the myocardium or going into a chamber, rather than extravasating into the pericardium. Echocardiography with administration of an intracoronary contrast agent (Definity, Lantheus Medical Imaging, North Billerica, MA) may better clarify if the perforation is actively extravasating and, if so, into what space. At the same time, it is important to remember that perforations that are hemodynamically stable may later degenerate, so ongoing monitoring and hypervigilance is paramount. Although most treatments needed to manage a perforation will occur during the index CTO PCI, delayed-onset tamponade can occur a few hours after the procedure, particularly with distal wire perforations, which may be bleeding slowly and are hard to detect. It should be noted that the absence of a perforation image throughout CTO PCI is not an absolute guarantee of not suffering tamponade in the immediate postprocedural period.[2] It is also important to always do an angiogram of the donor vessel at the end of the case to make sure that it has not been damaged and that no perforation is present.

On occasion, one will see what seems to be a coronary perforation in the distal aspect of a small vessel, but upon closer inspection, the "perforation" was present before the case. These coronary fistulas (arteriovenous or coronary cameral) can mimic perforation and are a reminder that sometimes reviewing the original angiograms may be helpful in determining whether or not a perforation has occurred.[12]

MANAGEMENT OF CORONARY PERFORATION

Approximately one-half of perforations occurring during CTO PCI will require treatment.[2,4] Perforation management depends on the perforation site, the severity of the perforation, and the hemodynamic status of the patients. As the operator, it is important to move quickly but to stay calm, work systematically, and communicate clearly. You will want to have the initial steps of perforation management at the forefront of your mind so you can execute swiftly. The staff also needs to be able to move quickly. As a drill to check the readiness of your laboratory, you can suddenly call out for a STAT pericardiocentesis kit (when you do not really need one) to see how quickly this emergency step is executed.

The first step in the management of a perforation is to inflate a balloon to stop, or at least slow, the bleeding. The balloon to artery ratio should be approximately 1.0 and the balloon may be inflated proximal to or at the site of

perforation (blocking balloon). In the case of a small distal vessel perforation, a microcatheter placed distally in the vessel can be put to suction. Alternatively, if a microcatheter has been clearly advanced outside of a vessel, leaving it there until definitive plans for treatment are made may prevent blood loss, and if there is blood loss into the pericardium, it can be withdrawn through the microcatheter. Taking the initial step of inflating a balloon or putting a microcatheter to suction will generally help stabilize the situation and provide time to determine what needs to be done next. This step may actually be all the treatment that is needed, but you still want to quickly prepare for your next steps. Intravenous fluids and vasopressors may be necessary to prevent or treat hypotension. Depending on the acuity of the situation, you will either want to perform a pericardiocentesis or get the pericardiocentesis kit ready, call for a stat echocardiogram, and notify others that you need (or may need) help. These could be a colleague to lend a hand and/or the surgical team if the perforation is severe and unlikely to respond to percutaneous treatment.

If, after a prolonged balloon inflation (up to 30 minutes depending on the patient's tolerance), the bleeding continues, a more definitive treatment will need to be pursued. If the perforation is in a large vessel, this situation will typically be managed with a covered stent. A perforation in a small, more distal vessel will typically be managed with embolization (coils, autologous fat, thrombin, microspheres or beads, gelfoam, thrombus, distal tip of a coronary wire, or silk sutures). If embolization is not feasible, another option is to put a covered stent in the main vessel that excludes the perforated small vessel.

Covered Stents

There are 2 covered stents available in the United States. The traditional covered stent that was approved by the US Food and Drug Administration (FDA) in January 2001 is the Jostent Graftmaster (Abbott Vascular, Santa Clara, CA). The newer covered stent, which became FDA approved in September 2018, is the Papyrus (Biotronik, Berlin, Germany). Although both devices are approved by the FDA, they remain under a humanitarian device exemption, which means that institutional review board approval must be obtained before use.

The Graftmaster has a polytetrafluoroethylene covering sandwiched between 2 stainless steel stent layers. It is intended for vessels 2.75 mm or larger and comes in 5 diameters

(2.8 mm, 3.5 mm, 4.0 mm, 4.5 mm, and 4.8 mm) and 3 lengths (16 mm, 19 mm, and 26 mm). The 2.8 mm to 4.0 mm stents can be delivered through a 6F guide, while the 4.5 mm and 4.8 mm require a 7F guide. The Papyrus is a cobalt chromium stent with a polyurethane covering on the abluminal side. It comes in 6 diameters (2.5 mm, 3.0 mm, 3.5 mm, 4.0 mm, 4.5 mm, and 5.0 mm) and 3 lengths (15 mm, 20 mm, and 26 mm). The 2.5 mm to 4.0 mm stents are 5F compatible, while the 4.5 mm and 5.0 mm stents require a 6F guide. Because of its single stent layer design and thinner stent struts (60 μm), the Papyrus has a smaller crossing profile and has been reported to be more flexible and deliverable than the Graftmaster. A systematic review of 29 studies involving 725 patients found no difference in target lesion revascularization, stent thrombosis, in-stent restenosis, or mortality between the 2 stents, although there seemed to be lower rates of pericardiocentesis or tamponade and emergency coronary artery bypass grafting with the Papyrus stent.[13] This finding suggests that, although the 2 stents may have a similar long-term safety profile, the Papyrus stent may offer better periprocedural outcomes, perhaps because of faster deliverability.[14]

There are several possible ways to deliver the covered stent. If the patient is relatively stable, the covered stent may be delivered through the same guide that was used for the prolonged balloon inflation. In this scenario, the balloon is deflated and removed, and the covered stent is advanced and deployed over the same coronary wire. If the patient does not tolerate having the balloon deflated for the time needed to deliver the stent, another option is to advance a guide extension that can block the perforation while the balloon is removed and the stent is delivered. If this procedure is insufficient, and the guide catheter is large enough, the covered stent can be delivered on a separate coronary wire alongside the blocking balloon through a single guide (block and deliver technique), deflating the balloon only briefly enough to remove it and its coronary wire before deploying the stent. Alternatively, a second guide catheter can be used to deliver the covered stent alongside the blocking balloon (ping-pong technique), again deflating the balloon only briefly enough to remove it and its coronary wire before deploying the stent. The disadvantage of these latter options is that the original wire will need to be removed and it may be in a location that you were hoping to maintain. These techniques for delivering covered stents can also be applied to the delivery of a microcatheter for embolization.

In addition to higher rates of stent thrombosis, a potential downside of covered stents is occlusion of the major side branches. If the covered stent needs to be deployed in a location that also crosses a side branch that you want to save, the covered stent can be fenestrated with a penetrative coronary wire, such as an Astato XS 20 (Asahi Intecc, Aichi, Japan), optionally with the help of a dual lumen microcatheter. Once the wire has penetrated the covered stent, it can be de-escalated to a less penetrative wire, followed by balloon inflation(s) and further stenting, if needed.[15,16]

Embolization

For smaller vessels that cannot be treated with a covered stent, embolization is generally the treatment of choice. There are multiple materials that can be used for embolization, including coils, autologous fat, thrombin, microspheres or beads, gelfoam, thrombus, the distal tip of a coronary wire, and silk sutures.

Coils are permanent metallic (stainless steel or platinum) agents with a wired structure of synthetic wool or Dacron fibers and thrombogenic properties. In coronary arteries, coils are generally delivered through a microcatheter (usually 0.018 inch, although there are some that can be delivered through an 0.014 inch device) that has been advanced to the location of interest. Coils are either pushable or detachable. With the pushable coils, you simply push them out the end of the microcatheter, whereas with the detachable coils, if you do not like the location or the way they are laying, they can be retrieved and redirected. Once they are in the desired position, they are detached. Coils come in a range of sizes (based on the loop diameter and the length), although there are limited coils to fit small coronary vessels. One will typically choose a loop diameter that is slightly larger that the target vessel to ensure complete vessel coverage. If the coil is too large, however, it may not go as distally as desired. The number of coils delivered will depend on how efficiently the coils are resulting in embolization of the vessel.

Autologous fat for embolization can be harvested from the abdominal or groin area (whether or not the patient had femoral access).[17] Several fat globules (≤1 mm in size) are placed into the proximal hub of a microcatheter that has been flushed with saline. The hub is then turned upside down and the fat will float into the hub toward the microcatheter lumen. This process can be aided by an introducer needle, if needed. Because fat is not visible on radiographs, the fat can be coated with contrast and/or the fat can be injected with diluted contrast to inform delivery. This process can be repeated as needed for complete hemostasis.

Thrombin is supplied as a sterile powder that is reconstituted with a diluent (generally nonheparinized saline). A small amount of thrombin (200–300 units) is injected slowly through a microcatheter to the desired site. The thrombin can be mixed with contrast to allow for angiographic visualization within the perforated segment. It is important not to get thrombin in the main vessel, so a small amount of air (<0.5 mL) can be injected after delivery to prevent backflow. Alternatively, if the vessel is large enough, the thrombin may be delivered through an inflated over-the-wire balloon to prevent reflux. Before removal, the microcatheter or balloon is flushed with a small amount of normal saline to clear any residual air and/or thrombin from the lumen. The microcatheter is then withdrawn quickly.[18,19] Thrombin can also be mixed with autologous blood to make a thrombin clot, or the thrombus itself can be used for embolization.

Microspheres (or beads) are spherical, hydrophilic, nonabsorbable particles that come in sizes ranging from 1 to 1500 microns (usually 300–700 microns for coronaries) and can be delivered through a microcatheter. They are made of various materials depending on the distributer and are mixed with contrast for visualization. As mentioned elsewhere in this article, several other materials can be used to embolize a vessel, but would generally only be used if the more standard materials are unavailable. There are also novel techniques for treating a perforation, such as using antegrade or retrograde dissection reentry to create a subintimal flap that can seal the site of perforation.[20]

Treatment of an epicardial collateral perforation deserves extra mention because the activated clotting time is generally high in these cases (approximately 300–350 seconds) and if the CTO has been recanalized, the collateral vessel will need to be sealed from both the donating and receiving directions. In addition, when injecting any embolization material into 1 side of an epicardial collateral, extreme care needs to be taken to not let that material go out the other end. For any collateral perforation (epicardial or septal), it should be noted that, if the CTO has not been opened, embolization of the collateral might lead to ischemia or infarction of the myocardial territory supplied by the collateral, unless additional collaterals exist.

Reversal of heparin may improve outcomes with CTO perforation, but must be delayed until after all intracoronary equipment is removed to prevent potential vessel thrombosis. Dosing of protamine is usually 20 to 25 mg intravenously. Whether a test dose is needed is unclear, but it should be noted that rapid infusions of protamine can cause hypotension, and other adverse effects include anaphylaxis and noncardiogenic pulmonary edema.

Prevention

Although not always possible, efforts to prevent coronary perforation in the first place are optimal. These include not performing ad hoc CTO PCI, using preprocedural coronary computed tomography angiography to delineate the proximal cap and/or vessel course when these are ambiguous on invasive angiography, always having dual catheters and performing orthogonal views to confirm wire location before advancing gear, de-escalating wires as soon as possible, using intravascular imaging to appropriately size equipment, and finally, not performing procedures that are beyond your training (such as using epicardial collaterals) without having a proctor available or the ability to effectively handle a perforation should it arise.

SUMMARY

Coronary perforation is a relatively common and potentially lethal complication of CTO PCI. Only about one-half of all perforations require treatment, and there are certain features that can signify a more high-risk perforation (Ellis type III, epicardial collateral location), but ultimately any perforation can be life threatening, and all perforations should be taken seriously. If a perforation occurs, the first step is to inflate a balloon (or put a microcatheter to suction) to stop the bleeding and plan for a more definitive treatment, if needed. In large vessels, this will generally involve a covered stent, whereas for smaller and/or more distal vessels, this will usually involve embolization. Because there are certain mechanisms known to increase the risk of perforation (such as overdilation, ploymer jacketed or penetrative wire exiting a vessel, or equipment advanced on a wire that is not on the vessel architecture), steps to minimize these occurrences in the fist place are best.

DISCLOSURE

J.A. Tremmel has received honorarium from Terumo, Boston Scientific, and Philips.

REFERENCES

1. Parsh J, Seth M, Green J, et al. Coronary artery perforations after contemporary percutaneous coronary interventions: evaluation of incidence, risk factors, outcomes, and predictors of mortality. Catheter Cardiovasc Interv 2017;89(6):966–73.
2. Azzalini L, Poletti E, Ayoub M, et al. Coronary artery perforation during chronic total occlusion percutaneous coronary intervention: epidemiology, mechanisms, management, and outcomes. EuroIntervention 2019;15(9):e804–11.
3. Danek BA, Karatasakis A, Tajti P, et al. Incidence, treatment, and outcomes of coronary perforation during chronic total occlusion percutaneous coronary intervention. Am J Cardiol 2017;120(8):1285–92.
4. Hirai T, Nicholson WJ, Sapontis J, et al. A detailed analysis of perforations during chronic total occlusion angioplasty. JACC Cardiovasc Interv 2019;12(19):1902–12.
5. Kinnaird T, Kwok CS, Kontopantelis E, et al. Incidence, determinants, and outcomes of coronary perforation during percutaneous coronary intervention in the United Kingdom Between 2006 and 2013: an analysis of 527 121 cases from the British cardiovascular intervention society database. Circ Cardiovasc Interv 2016;9(8):e003449.
6. Patel VG, Brayton KM, Tamayo A, et al. Angiographic success and procedural complications in patients undergoing percutaneous coronary chronic total occlusion interventions: a weighted meta-analysis of 18,061 patients from 65 studies. JACC Cardiovasc Interv 2013;6(2):128–36.
7. Wu K, Huang Z, Zhong Z, et al. Predictors, treatment, and long-term outcomes of coronary perforation during retrograde percutaneous coronary intervention via epicardial collaterals for recanalization of chronic coronary total occlusion. Catheter Cardiovasc Interv 2019;93(S1):800–9.
8. Ellis SG, Ajluni S, Arnold AZ, et al. Increased coronary perforation in the new device era. Incidence, classification, management, and outcome. Circulation 1994;90(6):2725–30.
9. Abdel-Karim AR, Vo M, Main ML, et al. Interventricular septal hematoma and coronary-ventricular fistula: a complication of retrograde chronic total occlusion intervention. Case Rep Cardiol 2016;2016:8750603.
10. Hashidomi H, Saito S. Dilation of the septal collateral artery and subsequent cardiac tamponade during retrograde percutaneous coronary intervention using a microcatheter for chronic total occlusion. J Interv Cardiol 2011;24(1):73–6.
11. Matsumi J, Adachi K, Saito S. A unique complication of the retrograde approach in angioplasty for chronic total occlusion of the coronary artery. Catheter Cardiovasc Interv 2008;72(3):371–8.
12. Kim TO, Koo HJ, Lee CW. Coronary arteriovenous fistulas mimicking coronary perforation after chronic total occlusion recanalization. Korean Circ J 2020;50(5):464–7.
13. Nagaraja V, Schwarz K, Moss S, et al. Outcomes of patients who undergo percutaneous coronary intervention with covered stents for coronary perforation: a systematic review and pooled analysis of data. Catheter Cardiovasc Interv 2019. https://doi.org/10.1002/ccd.28646.
14. Hernandez-Enriquez M, Lairez O, Campelo-Parada F, et al. Outcomes after use of covered stents to treat coronary artery perforations. Comparison of old and new-generation covered stents. J Interv Cardiol 2018;31(5):617–23.
15. Adusumalli S, Gaikwad N, Raffel C, et al. Treatment of rotablation-induced ostial left circumflex perforation by papyrus covered stent and its fenestration to recover the left anterior descending artery during CHIP procedure. Catheter Cardiovasc Interv 2019;93(6):E331–6.
16. Werner GS, Ahmed WH. Fenestration of a Papyrus PK covered stent to recover the occluded left main bifurcation after sealing a left main perforation during a CTO procedure. Cardiovasc Revasc Med 2017;18(6S1):41–4.
17. Shemisa K, Karatasakis A, Brilakis ES. Management of guidewire-induced distal coronary perforation using autologous fat particles versus coil embolization. Catheter Cardiovasc Interv 2017;89(2):253–8.
18. Fischell TA, Moualla SK, Mannem SR. Intracoronary thrombin injection using a microcatheter to treat guidewire-induced coronary artery perforation. Cardiovasc Revasc Med 2011;12(5):329–33.
19. Kotsia AP, Brilakis ES, Karmpaliotis D. Thrombin injection for sealing epicardial collateral perforation during chronic total occlusion percutaneous coronary interventions. J Invasive Cardiol 2014;26(9):E124–6.
20. Xenogiannis I, Tajti P, Nicholas Burke M, et al. An alternative treatment strategy for large vessel coronary perforations. Catheter Cardiovasc Interv 2019;93(4):635–8.

Perforation Mechanisms, Risk Stratification, and Management in the Post-Coronary Artery Bypass Grafting Patient

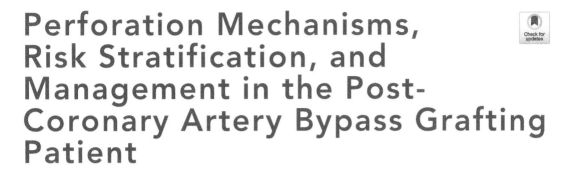

Taishi Hirai, MD[a],*, J. Aaron Grantham, MD[b,c]

KEYWORDS
• Chronic total occlusion • Percutaneous coronary intervention • Perforation • Coronary artery bypass grafting • Risk stratification

KEY POINTS
• Patients with prior history of coronary artery bypass grafting (CABG) with perforations during chronic total occlusion percutaneous coronary intervention are at higher risk of major adverse events compared with patients without history of CABG.
• Perforations in patients with prior CABG can have atypical presentation due to loculated pericardial effusions.
• The operators should avoid all unnecessary perforations and should be well prepared to treat perforations efficiently and effectively when it occurs.

 Video content accompanies this article at http://www.interventional.theclinics.com.

INTRODUCTION

Perforation is the most frequent major complication during chronic total occlusion percutaneous coronary intervention (CTO PCI). The incidence of coronary perforation in CTO PCI is 1.4% to 8.9%,[1,2] significantly higher than the incidence of perforation in non-CTO PCI (0.21%–0.71%).[3–5] In the OPEN CTO study, which enrolled 1000 consecutive patients from 12 leading centers in the United States and systematically used angiographic core laboratory and events adjudication, all 9 (0.9%) in-hospital deaths were associated with perforation.

Patients with prior coronary artery bypass grafting (CABG) accounted for half (44.4%) of all perforation-related deaths in OPEN. Therefore, the consequences of perforation in this subgroup seem uniquely dire. Whether this represents a vulnerable subgroup in CTO PCI due to complex anatomy, advanced disease, or unique management difficulty when perforations occur remains unclear. However, an understanding of the mechanisms, potential risk stratification strategies, and management of perforations during CTO PCI, with a specific focus on the patients with prior CABG, a particularly high-risk group, may help new operators to triage higher risk patients and advanced operators to prepare their teams and patients for challenging treatment decisions in CTO PCI.

[a] University of Missouri, One Hospital Drive, Columbia, MO 65212, USA; [b] Saint Luke's Mid America Heart Institute, 4401 Wornall Road, CV Research 9th floor, Kansas City, MO 64111, USA; [c] University of Missouri-Kansas City, Kansas City, MO, USA
* Corresponding author.
E-mail address: hirait@health.missouri.edu

Intervent Cardiol Clin 10 (2021) 101–107
https://doi.org/10.1016/j.iccl.2020.08.001
2211-7458/21/© 2020 Elsevier Inc. All rights reserved.

Mechanisms of Perforation

The main perforation mechanisms in general are large vessel perforation such as vessel rupture after stenting and distal perforations from guidewire exit or device advancement through a wire exit. There are other mechanisms of perforations to consider specifically in patients with prior CABG. First, degenerated or occluded vein grafts that are often used as a retrograde conduit are friable and at higher risk of graft rupture or perforation. Graft rupture can occur when crossing the occluded grafts or during balloon inflation. Guidewire exits in bypass grafts are harder to identify, as there is no way to evaluate the wire position in an occluded graft. In other words, the wire and vessel "dance," a sign that the guidewire is moving with the vessel architecture during a retrograde injection, which typically can be used to assess the wire position in a native vessel, is not possible. Graft rupture can also occur when ballooning the graft, such as when advancing the guide-extension over an anchored balloon. Secondly, the anastomosis sites are often challenging to cross, due to the suture line or vessel deformity or "tenting." Use of laser device or use of knuckled stiffer guidewires and Carlino technique (selective injection of contrast through the microcatheter) is often necessary in this setting, and these techniques are inherently at higher risk of perforation. Finally, as patients with prior coronary artery bypass surgery (CABG) often have more complex anatomy compared with patients without prior CABG, use of epicardial collateral channels can be enticing. However, as discussed earlier, epicardial perforations in patients with prior CABG are high risk of adverse outcomes, and these vessels should be avoided if possible and attempted only by the most experienced operators.

Risk Stratification

Preprocedural planning

CTO operators should assess patient-related factors associated with perforations and apply strategies to mitigate the risk of perforations.

Patient-related factors. Patient-related factors such as older age, female sex, previous history of CABG, and complex anatomy with higher J-CTO score are associated with increased risk of perforation.[2,6] In patients with higher risk of perforation, more careful assessment of risk and benefit of the CTO PCI is necessary. Specifically, less-experienced operators starting a CTO program may consider referring the high-risk patient to a more experienced operator. To improve the triage of the complex patients to

operators with appropriate skillsets, development of perforation-specific risk-stratification tool could be useful and requires further study.

Local factors and expertise of the operator and staff in cardiac catheterization laboratory. Having necessary equipment to treat perforations in the cardiac catheterization laboratory is fundamental for a CTO program. Similarly, CTO PCI should be performed at a center with surgical backup. The cardiac catheterization laboratory should be equipped with, at minimum, pericardiocentesis kit, covered stents, and embolization materials such as coil, thrombin, or microsphere. Furthermore, operator and the staff should have thorough experience to use these techniques and devices at emergent situations. Some experienced operators perform a drill for the staff to prepare for emergent situations, by calling for pericardiocentesis kit at a random timing.

Selection of strategies. Although retrograde techniques have reported to be associated with an increase in adverse outcomes,[7,8] recent study suggests that this association could be explained by the complexity of the lesion itself, as retrograde techniques are applied more often in patients with challenging anatomy.[9] Although this finding highlights the importance of using both antegrade and retrograde approach to maximize the efficiency and success rates of the procedure,[10] use of epicardial collateral may have a unique risk profile. This risk profile was highlighted by the finding that the epicardial collateral perforations were associated with significantly higher mortality compared with other locations, such as large vessel or septal perforators.[9] Therefore, experienced operators may select subintimal tracking and re-entry with staged stenting or subintimal plaque modification with repeat attempt over high-risk epicardial collaterals in some selected situations.[11–13] Details of these techniques are discussed in another chapter. Whether these techniques are associated with less perforations and adverse outcomes compared with epicardial collateral crossing requires further study.

Intraprocedure

Perforation avoidance/early recognition. The operator should practice basic techniques to prevent perforations, as summarized in Box 1. These strategies include exchanging CTO-specific guidewires for workhorse guidewires immediately after lesion crossing, minimizing the use of higher-risk guidewires (stiffer tapered wires) and deescalating to safer guidewires, and

> **Box 1**
> **Perforation avoidance strategies**
>
> During lesion crossing
>
> 1. When using stiff wire for antegrade strategy, monitor wire position in 2 perpendicular views ("dancing sign").
> 2. Once proximal cap is crossed, "de-escalate" the guidewire to a softer guidewire.
> 3. Meticulous attention of the wire position. If the guidewire is outside the vessel, or in a small side branch, do not advance the balloon or microcatheter.
> 4. Recognition of the position of CrossBoss microcatheter to avoid side-branch exit.
> 5. Consider dissection re-entry with knuckle guidewire rather than attempting wiring of a long lesion.
>
> During collateral crossing:
>
> 1. Avoid excessive force to the microcatheter when it is not crossing the collateral channel.
> 2. Protect the collateral channel with microcatheter when removing the externalized guidewire.
>
> After lesion crossing:
>
> 1. Immediately exchange the speciality wire to workhorse guidewire.
> 2. Confirmation of the re-entry to true lumen.
> 3. Aggressive atherectomy for eccentric calcification.
> 4. Moderate pressure postdilation in subintimal space inflation ($\sim$14 atm if in subinitimal space especially in eccentric calcified vessel).

meticulous attention to the guidewire relationship to vessel architecture. It is also important for the operators to recognize the guidewire exiting the vessel and not to follow the guidewire with a device. Long cine run should be performed at the completion of the case to screen for small and distal perforations. Details of these issues are covered in the previous chapter.

In regard to the patients with previous CABG it should be noted that perforations can result in bleeding into unusual spaces. As an example, many post-CABG patients have occluded bypass grafts that once subtended the CTO target vessel. These occluded grafts can be used as retrograde conduits and are, in many instances, safer than epicardial collaterals. However, given the friable and thin wall of the vein grafts, the authors recommend generally avoiding knuckled guidewires when crossing these occluded grafts.

In addition, operators must realize that perforation of these grafts can result in bleeding into the mediastinum.[14] Mediastinal bleeding cannot be seen routinely with echocardiography. Therefore, when using old venous bypass grafts, it is important to take a final injection in the graft, perform CT scanning in patients with suspected graft perforations, and have a low threshold for sealing graft perforations.

Management

Even the most careful CTO operator will experience perforations. When it occurs, the operator should be prepared to triage and treat the perforation effectively in a timely fashion. The main goal is to avoid the major adverse outcomes associated with perforation such as cardiac tamponade, myocardial infarction, or death.

Once the perforation is recognized, it is important for the operator to risk-stratify the lesion. The operator should avoid excessive injection once the perforation is identified and assess the hemodynamics and symptoms of the patient. Ellis criteria has been used traditionally to classify the angiographic findings of the perforation (**Box 2**). Compared with class I and class II perforations, class III perforations are associated with higher incidence of dramatic complications.[4] However, it is important to note that this classification system was established at a prestent, angioplasty era in a cohort of patients undergoing non-CTO PCI, and therefore its use may be limited in CTO cases.

In a more contemporary study in patients with CTO PCI, the perforation that was associated with major adverse outcomes was larger in size, more often at a proximal or collateral location, and had high-risk shape, which was defined as "cloud-like" and "floating" (**Fig. 1**).[9] Importantly among the 8 perforations that occurred in epicardial collateral vessel, 4 patients suffered inpatient mortality.[9] These findings suggest that perforations that are larger in size, in proximal location, or with high-risk shape require treatment. Furthermore, the perforation of epicardial collateral location should be treated regardless of size as Ellis criteria likely do not apply. An example of an epicardial perforation of a patient who suffered in-hospital mortality from the OPEN CTO study is presented in **Fig. 2** (see also **Video 3**). It highlights that even small size epicardial perforation can cause devastating outcome.

Most importantly, patients with previous CABG can present with loculated effusion, which is much more challenging to diagnose and treat. It may be difficult to diagnose due to absence of classic signs of tamponade physiology such as pulsus pradoxus or Kussmaul sign. They could also have delayed presentation and become hemodynamically unstable after having stable hemodynamics and transferred out of the cardiac catheterization laboratory. Furthermore, because of the atypical location (mediastinum), it may be challenging to visualize the hematoma or loculated effusion by echocardiogram. In these situations, CT scan could be helpful for diagnosis.

Few patterns of atypical presentation are summarized as follows:

1. Atrial and ventricular compression
   The compression can occur at right atrial, left atrial, right ventricle, or left ventricle level. All can be hemodynamically significant through compression and dysfunction.
   Left atrial compression seems to be more common when perforation occurred in right ventricular marginal branch or apical branches from LCx or right coronary artery (RCA) or atrioventricular groove collateral vessels. Patients can present with similar physiology with mitral

stenosis. On the other hand, loculated effusion that compresses the right side of the heart can occur with perforation of RCA. When there is right ventricular outflow tract obstruction the patient can present with similar physiology with pulmonic stenosis.[15]

2. Hemothorax
   In a rare occasion, bleeding from perforation in a patient with previous CABG can connect directly to the thoracic cavity and develop left hemothorax.[16] This will be important to recognize, as patient may present with hemorrhagic shock due to the large amount of blood loss, compared with obstructive shock that is often seen in patient with cardiac tamponade.

TREATMENT STRATEGY

The treatment strategy of perforation in general is discussed in detail in the previous chapter. In brief, treatment strategies include prolonged balloon inflation, pericardiocentesis, covered stent placement, and embolization.

In patients with prior CABG, appropriate recognition of loculated effusion is key and drainage of the effusion is often necessary (Fig. 3, see also Video 4). It may require ultrasound-guided approach from an atypical location, with computed tomography (CT) or transesophageal echocardiography guidance[17,18] or surgical evacuation.[19] When mediastinal bleeding from vein graft perforation is suspected, operators should have low threshold to perform additional testing with CT scan and have low threshold to seal the perforation. In case of wire perforation of vein grafts, the

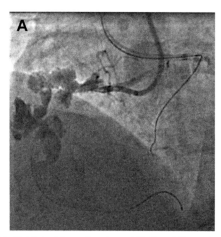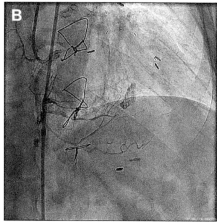

Fig. 1. (*A, B*) High-risk perforations. (*A*) Cloud-like. (*B*) Floating. See also Videos 1 and 2.

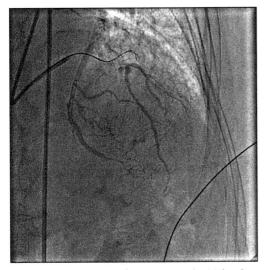

Fig. 2. An epicardial perforation. See also Video 3.

authors recommend thrombin administration as a first choice to seal the graft.

Covered Stent

Covered stents are often used to seal large vessel perforations. The PK Papyrus (Biotronik, Berlin, Germany) covered stent was introduced into the US market in 2018. This stent consists of a 90-um cover made of electrospun polyurethane that is mounted on a 60-um thin-strut stent. Compared with the traditional sandwich design (2 stents with polytetrafluoroethylene in between) of the older Graftmaster (Abbott Vascular, Abbott Park, IL), this stent is less bulky and therefore can be advanced through smaller diameter catheters with better crossability. Both devices are only available for use in the United States with the restrictions of a humanitarian device use exemption. These devices

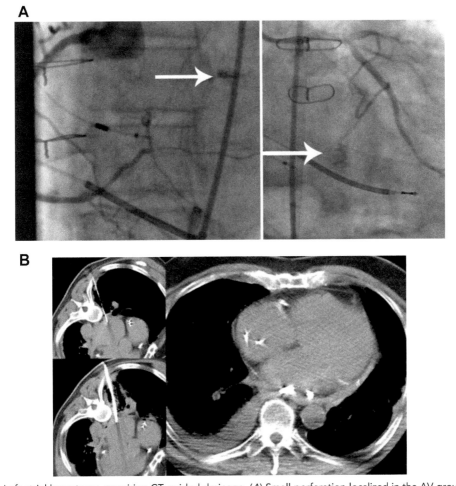

Fig. 3. Left atrial hematoma, requiring CT-guided drainage. (*A*) Small perforation localized in the AV grove (*white arrows*). (left, RCA injection; right, left coronary injection). (*B*) Percutaneous drainage of hematoma (left upper, needle aspiration; left lower, drain tube placement; right, resolution of pericardial hematoma). See also Video 4. (*From* Wilson WM, Spratt JC, Lombardi WL. Cardiovascular collapse post chronic total occlusion percutaneous coronary intervention due to a compressive left atrial hematoma managed with percutaneous drainage. Catheter Cardiovasc Interv 2015;86:407-11; with permission.)

require Institutional Review Board approval and detailed reporting of every use and should be mandatory in every laboratory performing coronary intervention, especially those performing CTO PCI.

Embolization/Thrombosis
Fat embolization
Fat embolization can be performed by harvesting the patient's fat from femoral sheath site. It is mixed in saline or contrast and pushed into the microcatheter with a needle introducer.

Thrombin
Thrombin is typically diluted to 100U/cc and will be given 2 to 3 cc (200–300U) at a time. It is important to dispose the microcatheter immediately and exchange the sterile gloves to avoid unwanted thrombus formation in the interventional system. The guide catheter must be back bled after thrombin administration. Thrombin is the preferred approach in sealing wire perforated grafts.

Coil embolization
There are many types of coils in the market but can be divided into pushable coils and detachable coils. Detachable coils are often preferred, as it can be repositioned until it is positioned at the optimal location. Some coils require larger microcatheter for deployment, and it is important to understand the compatibility of the coils and the microcatheters.

Gel foam
Gel foam is a product available in every surgical operating room. A small piece can be cut, rolled into a ball, placed in the hub of a microcatheter, dissolved in contrast, and then injected to occlude small wire perforations.

Heparin Reversal
Most experienced operators recommend reversing the heparin with protamine only after all equipment is removed from the vessel. Heparin reversal with indwelling equipment can cause device thrombosis, which can worsen the situation. It is also important to drain any hemodynamically significant pericardial effusion before heparin reversal, as it is extremely difficult to percutaneously remove clotted blood in the pericardium and may require emergent surgical removal. The clinical impact of clotted blood in the mediastinum is not known for certain but not thought to be significant.

SUMMARY

In conclusion, perforation in patients with prior CABG undergoing CTO PCI can cause dire consequences, possibly related to their complex anatomy and unique techniques applied during the procedure. It is important for the operators to avoid, appropriately identify, and treat the perforations in a timely fashion. Further study is necessary to understand the mechanism and better risk-stratify the perforations in this population.

Clinics care points

- Perforation is a most important complication of CTO PCI associated with high morbidity and mortality.
- The operators should avoid all unnecessary perforations and should be well prepared to treat perforations efficiently and effectively when it occurs.
- Patients with prior CABG have increased risk of perforation and are at higher risk of adverse outcomes possibly related to the atypical presentation and unique management difficulty.
- Loculated effusions may require drainage from atypical approach, CT-guided approach, or surgical evacuation.
- Epicardial perforation requires special attention and most likely requires treatment.
- Further study in better predicting perforations is necessary.

DISCLOSURE

T. Hirai: honoraria from Abiomed. J.A. Grantham: speaking fees and honoraria from Boston Scientific, Abbott Vascular, and Asahi Intecc and institutional research grant support from Boston Scientific. He is a part time employee of Corindus Vascular Robotics and own equity in the company.

SUPPLEMENTARY DATA

Supplementary data related to this article can be found online at https://doi.org/10.1016/j.iccl.2020.08.001.

REFERENCES

1. Sapontis J, Salisbury AC, Yeh RW, et al. Early procedural and health status outcomes after chronic total occlusion angioplasty: A report from the

OPEN-CTO Registry (Outcomes, Patient Health Status, and Efficiency iN Chronic Total Occlusion Hybrid Procedures). JACC Cardiovasc Interv 2017; 10:1523–34.

2. Kinnaird T, Anderson R, Ossei-Gerning N, et al. Legacy effect of coronary perforation complicating percutaneous coronary intervention for chronic total occlusive disease: An analysis of 26 807 cases from the British Cardiovascular Intervention Society Database. Circ Cardiovasc Interv 2017;10:e004642.

3. Al-Lamee R, Ielasi A, Latib A, et al. Incidence, predictors, management, immediate and long-term outcomes following grade III coronary perforation. JACC Cardiovasc Interv 2011;4:87–95.

4. Hendry C, Fraser D, Eichhofer J, et al. Coronary perforation in the drug-eluting stent era: incidence, risk factors, management and outcome: the UK experience. Eurointervention 2012;8:79–86.

5. Lemmert ME, van Bommel RJ, Diletti R, et al. Clinical Characteristics and Management of Coronary Artery Perforations: A Single-Center 11-Year Experience and Practical Overview. J Am Heart Assoc 2017;6:e007049.

6. Danek BA, Karatasakis A, Tajti P, et al. Incidence, treatment, and outcomes of coronary perforation during chronic total occlusion percutaneous coronary intervention. Am J Cardiol 2017;120:1285–92.

7. Karmpaliotis D, Karatasakis A, Alaswad K, et al. Outcomes with the use of the retrograde approach for coronary chronic total occlusion interventions in a contemporary multicenter US registry. Circ Cardiovasc Interv 2016;9:e003434.

8. Stetler J, Karatasakis A, Christakopoulos GE, et al. Impact of crossing technique on the incidence of periprocedural myocardial infarction during chronic total occlusion percutaneous coronary intervention. Catheter Cardiovasc Interv 2016;88:1–6.

9. Hirai T, Nicholson WJ, Sapontis J, et al. A detailed analysis of perforations during chronic total occlusion angioplasty. JACC Cardiovasc Interv 2019;12:1902–12.

10. Brilakis ES, Grantham JA, Rinfret S, et al. A percutaneous treatment algorithm for crossing coronary chronic total occlusions. JACC Cardiovasc Interv 2012;5:367–79.

11. Hirai T, Grantham JA, Sapontis J, et al. Impact of subintimal plaque modification procedures on health status after unsuccessful chronic total occlusion angioplasty. Catheter Cardiovasc Interv 2018; 91:1035–42.

12. Goleski PJ, Nakamura K, Liebeskind E, et al. Revascularization of coronary chronic total occlusions with subintimal tracking and reentry followed by deferred stenting: Experience from a high-volume referral center. Catheter Cardiovasc Interv 2019; 93:191–8.

13. Hirai T, Grantham JA, Gosch KL, et al. Impact of subintimal or plaque modification on repeat chronic total occlusion angioplasty following an unsuccessful attempt. JACC Cardiovasc Interv 2020; 13:1010–2.

14. Wyderka R, Adamowicz J, Nowicki P, et al. Perforation of saphenous vein graft with mediastinal haemorrhage leading to near closure of distal graft segment. SAGE Open Med Case Rep 2019;7. 2050313X19838745.

15. Kawase Y, Hayase M, Ito S, et al. Compression of right ventricular out-flow due to localized hematoma after coronary perforation during PCI. Catheter Cardiovasc Interv 2003;58:202–6.

16. Frangieh AH, Klainguti M, Luscher TF, et al. Left-sided haemothorax after iatrogenic coronary perforation in a patient with prior bypass surgery. Eur Heart J 2015;36:128.

17. Wilson WM, Spratt JC, Lombardi WL. Cardiovascular collapse post chronic total occlusion percutaneous coronary intervention due to a compressive left atrial hematoma managed with percutaneous drainage. Catheter Cardiovasc Interv 2015;86: 407–11.

18. Hashimoto Y, Inoue K. Endoscopic ultrasound-guided transesophageal pericardiocentesis: an alternative approach to a pericardial effusion. Endoscopy 2016;48(Suppl 1 UCTN):E71–2.

19. Krabatsch T, Becher D, Schweiger M, et al. Severe left atrium compression after percutaneous coronary intervention with perforation of a circumflex branch of the left coronary artery. Interact Cardiovasc Thorac Surg 2010;11:811–3.

Access Selection for Chronic Total Occlusion Percutaneous Coronary Intervention and Complication Management

Luiz F. Ybarra, MD, PhD, MBA[a],
Stéphane Rinfret, MD, SM, FRCP(C), FSCAI[b],*

KEYWORDS

- Chronic total occlusion • Percutaneous coronary intervention • Vascular access • Radial access
- Femoral access • Vascular complications

KEY POINTS

- Although femoral access is the traditional access to chronic total occlusion percutaneous coronary intervention, the use of the radial approach has been increasing significantly.
- Both accesses have advantages and disadvantages.
- The radial access has minimal clinical risks, but it is limited by the guiding catheter size and support to perform more complex techniques.
- The femoral access is associated with more vascular complications, but it must be used in more complex cases.
- Complication management is similar to what is done for regular percutaneous coronary intervention, although the risks can be slightly higher due the need of dual access.

INTRODUCTION

Access-site selection for chronic total occlusion (CTO) percutaneous coronary intervention (PCI) may be influenced by multiple factors, including physician practice and preference, anatomic variation, vessel occlusion or spasm, history of coronary artery bypass graft (CABG) surgery, planned initial revascularization strategy, and lesion complexity. Moreover, CTO PCI presents several additional access challenges compared with traditional PCI, including the need for multiple arterial accesses and large-caliber guide catheters (GCs), to fit the different dedicated devices and facilitate CTO techniques.

A recent meta-analysis showed that CTO PCI technical success is similar with both radial artery (RA) and femoral artery (FA) accesses,[1] which corroborates the findings of other large series.[2–5] Although it is reassuring that most cases can be performed by both accesses, the careful reader/operator realizes that these results likely were subject to selection bias.[6] Identifying when each of these accesses should be used, along with their specific advantages and disadvantages (Table 1), is of paramount importance to achieve such high CTO PCI success rates, while minimizing complications and maximizing bailout options.

[a] London Health Sciences Centre, Schulich School of Medicine & Dentistry, Western University, 339 Windermere Road, Room B6-127, London, Ontario N6A 5A5, Canada; [b] Division of Cardiology, Department of Medicine, McGill University, McGill University Health Centre, Glen Site, 1001 Boulevard Décarie, Montreal, Quebec H4A 3J1, Canada
* Corresponding author.
E-mail address: stephane.rinfret@mcgill.ca
Twitter: @YbarraLuiz (L.F.Y.); @RinfretStephane (S.R.)

Intervent Cardiol Clin 10 (2021) 109–120
https://doi.org/10.1016/j.iccl.2020.09.009
2211-7458/21/© 2020 Elsevier Inc. All rights reserved.

Table 1 Advantages and disadvantages of the radial and femoral accesses			
Pros and Cons		**Radial**	**Femoral**
Advantages	Clinical	• Early sitting • Early ambulation • Improved patient comfort • Less major bleeding • Less vascular complications • Less transfusion • Potential decrease in in-hospital mortality	• Less risk of artery occlusion • Use for mechanical circulatory support in high-risk patients
	Procedural	• Earlier discharge • Lower cost • Retrograde catheter for most cases	• Allows larger catheters • Increased catheter support • Minimal impact of guiding catheter position with inspiration/expiration • Better for ostial CTOs • All CTO PCI techniques can be performed
Similarities		• Similar rates of technical success, especially in less complex procedures • Similar risk of procedural complication • Similar in-hospital MACE	
Disadvantages	Clinical	• Higher risk of artery occlusion	• Higher risk of major bleeding • Higher risk for transfusion • Higher risk of vascular access complications • Higher risk of adverse outcomes if access-site complication occurs • Possible higher risk of in-hospital mortality
	Procedural	• Use of larger guiding catheters is limited • Less support • Inspiration/expiration impacts guiding catheter position • Not ideal for ostial CTOs • Left radial: uncomfortable for the operator	• None

The objective of this article is to present a rationale for access selection for CTO PCI and to briefly discuss complication management in case it occurs.

FEMORAL ACCESS

FA has been the traditional access for CTO PCI for many years. A large British registry of CTO PCIs performed between 2006 and 2013 showed that, although its use has been significantly decreasing over time, FA still was used in 68.2% of the cases.[5] Another registry reporting more contemporary data showed that at least 1 FA was used in 80% of the cases.[3]

Advantages
Due to its caliber, the FA can accommodate larger (8F or higher) GCs compared with the RA. These catheters allow for the use of simultaneous microcatheters, facilitating complex antegrade maneuvers (Table 2), and providing increased passive support compared with smaller ones. The FA size also

Table 2
Compatibility of chronic total occlusion percutaneous coronary intervention techniques with different guiding catheters

	5 French	6 French	7 French	8 French
Internal diameter (in)	0.56–0.58	0.70–0.71	0.78–0.81	0.88–0.90
External diameter at the arterial access site (mm)	2.3	2.52–2.60	2.85–3.10	3.20–3.50
Parallel wire technique (antegrade CTO PCI technique)				
Wire + 1 microcatheter	Y	Y	Y	Y
2 microcatheters	N	Y	Y	Y
1 microcatheter + 1 OTW balloon	N	N	Y	Y
2 OTW balloons	N	N	N	Y
Side-branch anchoring balloon and balloon trapping (useful for both antegrade and retrograde CTO PCI techniques)				
1 monorail balloon + 1 microcatheter	N	Y	Y	Y
1 monorail balloon + 1 OTW balloon	N	Y	Y	Y
CTO PCI: IVUS-guidance (useful for both antegrade and retrograde CTO PCI techniques)				
With simultaneous wire inside	Y	Y	Y	Y
With simultaneous microcatheter	N	N	Y	Y
Adjunctive devices (useful for both antegrade and retrograde CTO PCI techniques)				
Rotablator (Boston Scientific, Marlborough Massachusetts, USA) 1.25–1.75 mm burr	N	Y	Y	Y
Rotablator 2.0–2.25 mm burr	N	N	Y	Y
Laser 0.9–1.4 mm	Y	Y	Y	Y
Laser 1.7–2.2 mm	N	N	Y	Y
Tornus (Asahi Intecc, Seto-shi, Aichi, Japan) 2.1F	N	Y	Y	Y
Tornus 2.6F	N	Y	Y	Y
Corsair (Asahi Intecc, Seto-shi, Aichi, Japan)	N	Y	Y	Y
CrossBoss (Boston Scientific, Marlborough Massachusetts, USA) catheter	N	Y	Y	Y
Stingray LP balloon	N	Y (cannot trap)	Y	Y

Abbreviations: IVUS, intravascular ultrasound; N, No; OTW, over-the-wire; Y, Yes.
    From Burzotta F, De Vita M, Lefevre T, Tommasino A, Louvard Y, Trani C. Radial approach for percutaneous coronary interventions on chronic total occlusions: technical issues and data review. *Catheterization and cardiovascular interventions : official journal of the Society for Cardiac Angiography & Interventions.* 2014;83(1):47-57; with permission.

makes its less prone to occlusion compared with the RA.

The GC engagement in the coronary ostium is less affected by the inspiration and expiration movements when coming through the FA. This is of particular interest in anomalous coronary ostia and CTOs of the left main or right coronary arteries ostia. In these cases, the GC often cannot achieve a coaxial intubation, which makes it more unstable and less supportive and, therefore, less reliable (Fig. 1).

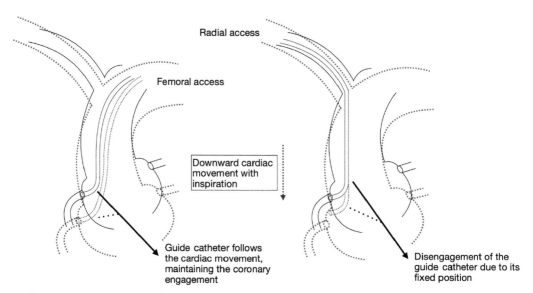

Fig. 1. GC behavior with inspiration according to access site.

The FA also can be used to accommodate a mechanical circulatory support in high-risk CTO PCI, although its use can be associated with hemorrhagic complications in up to two-thirds of the cases.[3]

Use of at least 1 FA is needed if a triple access is needed in a post-CABG case. In many post-CABG CTOs, collaterals come from multiple arteries or grafts. A typical example is treatment of a right coronary artery (RCA) CTO that receives collaterals not only from the native left anterior descending artery (LAD) and circumflex artery but also from the left internal mammary artery (LIMA)-LAD graft trough septal channels. The use of a triple-access eases visualization of the distal bed and helps clarify if there is presence or not of a connection between the posterolateral and the posterior descending artery. In such cases, 2 radials could be used: 1 for the LIMA GC and the other for the left main coronary artery GC, whereas the femoral access allows for the use of a very supportive 8F for the RCA. FA also should be privileged when using a left-sided saphenous vein graft (SVG) for retrograde access, because it increases support (Fig. 2).

Disadvantages

The main disadvantage of the FA access compared with the RA is its higher risk of major bleeding and vascular access complications.[1,3,5] A recent meta-analysis performed by Megaly and colleagues[1] showed that major bleeding occurred in 0.18% of the RA cases compared with 0.9% of the FA ones (odds ratio [OR] 0.22;

95% CI, 0.10–0.45; $P<.001$; $I^2 = 0$%) and that access-site complications occurred in 0.75% versus 1.79%, respectively (OR 0.34; 95% CI, 0.22–0.51; $P<.001$; I2 = 0%). An international CTO registry performed a relevant comparison of cases performed by RA and FA only and a combination of both (radial-femoral access [RA + FA]). It showed that major bleeding occurred in 0.55% of the RA cases compared with 1.94% of the FA cases and 0.88% of the combined RA + FA cases.[3] The location of the bleeding was the access site in 61.8% and a

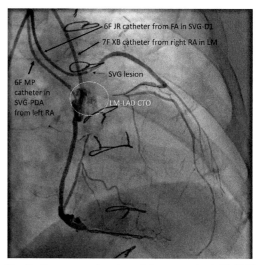

Fig. 2. Case example using triple access for LAD CTO PCI in a post-CABG patient. D1, first diagonal branch; JR, Judkins right; LM, left main coronary artery; MP, multipurpose; PDA, posterior descending artery.

majority of access-site bleeding complications occurred during RA + FA cases (61.9% of access-site bleedings), whereas one-third (33.3%) occurred with FA cases and only 4.8% with RA cases (P = .003). This likely was driven by the higher use of mechanical circulatory support devices in the combined group (65.2%) compared with FA (18.9%) and RA cases (14.3%) (P = .007). These already are known potential complications of FA compared with RA access in regular PCI, but it becomes more evident in the CTO PCI context due to the need of dual accesses, which increases the risk further.

Moreover, FA-site complications in CTO PCI are strongly predictive of adverse patient outcomes.[5] Kinnaird and colleagues[5] demonstrated that FA complications increased the likelihood of procedural coronary complications (adjusted OR 3.4; 95% CI, 2.4–4.8; P<.0001), postprocedural stroke (adjusted OR 16.5; 95% CI, 2.0–137.5; P<.0001), periprocedural myocardial infarction (adjusted OR 3.2; 95% CI, 1.2–8.7; P = .002), and in-hospital major bleeding (adjusted OR 28.9; 95% CI, 17.5–47.6; P<.0001). Studies also have shown that FA is associated with increased transfusions and short-term mortality.[1]

Strategies to minimize FA-site complications (aside from use of RA) includes routine fluoroscopy imaging, vascular ultrasound, and micropuncture kit, and these techniques in concert should become adopted more widely.[7]

RADIAL OR ULNAR ACCESS

RA became the default access for ACS patients after the publication of the RIVAL, RIFLE-STEACS, and STEMI-RADIAL trials.[8–10] After that, the RA was proved to improve outcomes not only in ACS patients but also the entire spectrum of patients with coronary artery disease.[11] Thus, the RA became the default approach for any coronary intervention and was adopted early in the CTO PCI field.[12]

The use of RA increased significantly from 2006 to 2013 (15.4% to 42.1%) according to the British registry.[5] Dual wrist access increased from 0% to 6.6% and dual wrist/femoral from 17% to 52.8% in the same time period. An international registry published by Tajti and colleagues[3] assessing data from 2012 to 2018 showed a more significant increase of RA use (11% to 67%).

One of the initial concerns of RA was on radiation exposure. The international registry, discussed previously, showed a significant decrease on overall procedure and fluoroscopy time, air kerma radiation dose, and even contrast volume.[3] Although this reduction also could be due to other factors, such as better machines, improved radiation protocols, increased and operator awareness, among others, it is reassuring to know that RA did not hinder this evolution.

Another misconception about the RA is that it may decrease success rates due to limits in GC size, especially in more complex CTOs. Tajti and colleagues[3] showed that RA and RA + FA had similar success rates compared with FA across the entire spectrum of J-CTO score. RA had higher success rates than FA in J-CTO score 4 and score 5 (87% vs 54%, respectively; P = .021, and 90% vs 68%, respectively; P = .04). Even though these results likely are secondary to selection bias, it is again reassuring that using the RA in selected complex anatomies does not have a negative impact in success rates.

The ulnar artery can be used as a feasible alternative access, although data in the CTO PCI field are lacking. A meta-analysis of 6 trials comparing ulnar access and RA showed similar incidence of major adverse cardiovascular events (MACEs), vascular complications, arterial access time, fluoroscopy time, and contrast load.[13] Kedev and colleagues[14] assessed the feasibility and safety of using the ulnar access when the radial was not available in 476 consecutive patients, with high success rates and low incidence of vascular complications. They also performed a subgroup analysis in 240 patients with documented ipsilateral RA occlusion (RAO) and showed that there was no difference in terms of procedural success and any vascular complication compared with those patients without radial occlusion. Despite this, when the RA clearly is occluded, the authors recommend not using the ulnar access until larger prospective data confirm safety. Moreover, the authors usually do not advocate for the use of ipsilateral radial and ulnar accesses for dual injection in CTO PCI, although 1 study showed its feasibility and safety in selected patients.[15]

Advantages

RA is known to improve patient comfort, especially after the procedure, decrease cost, and allow earlier discharge.[11,16] Specific to CTO PCI, the radial approach is perfect for retrograde injections, especially when there is no plan for retrograde crossing.[17] Dual radial approach also permits early sitting and ambulation, which can be a big advantage in some patients.

As discussed previously, RA also is associated with lower rates of major bleeding, lower risk of access-site complications,[1,3,5] and possible lower risk of in-hospital death.[1,5] Its use also should be maximized when a triple access is required (using both radials), to avoid the use of dual femoral.

Disadvantages

Most of the disadvantages of the RA comes from the limitations on GC size. In their article comparing RA and FA in CTO PCI, Tanaka and colleagues[2] conclude that albeit transradial CTO PCI may be feasible in simpler cases, complex CTOs are better managed from the femoral approach. A careful analysis of the groups' characteristics depicts a clear selection bias. When the RA was selected, GCs less than or equal to 6F were used in 91% of cases, whereas greater than or equal to 7F were used in greater than or equal to 95% of TA. Thus, this study actually was a comparison of small versus large GCs in the success of CTO PCI. Perhaps the conclusions would be similar if this study were done only using the FA and less than or equal to 6F versus greater than or equal to 7F GCs. Despite that, this study did confirm that RA has fewer vascular complications than FA.

Although several CTO PCI techniques can be done with 6F GCs using the miniaturized devices available nowadays, more complex cases require yet larger catheters. RA may limit the efficacy of the antegrade dissection and re-entry (ADR) technique if only a 6F GC can be used. With the advent of the 6F TrapLiner (Teleflex, Wayne, PA, USA) device (a guide-extension attached to a balloon), however, ADR now can be performed using the Stingray LP (low-profile balloon) (Boston Scientific, Marlborough, Massachusetts, USA) and maintain the ability to trap of the wire, an essential maneuver in CTO PCI.

Without the TrapLiner, the StingRay LP balloon can be exchanged only with guide wire extensions through 6F, making it more difficult and unreliable. Often the operator may be limited to perform noncontrolled ADR techniques, such as subintimal tracking and re-entry and limited antegrade subintimal tracking, which are known to have worst outcomes.[18]

The use of larger GCs, however, may increase the risk of radial occlusion[1] and also would be challenging in women with smaller RAs. To overcome limitation of radial size to accommodate an 8F sheath and catheter, Dautov and colleagues[19] described the effectiveness of a home-made 8F sheathless system to be used transradially (Fig. 3). An alternative to the long

dilator of the 6F Flexor® Shuttle® Guiding Sheath (Cook Medical, Bloomington, IN, USA) is the use of a 6F Slip-Cath Beacon Tip Hydrophilic Catheter (Cook Medical, Bloomington, IN, USA) angiographic catheter, as displayed in Fig. 3. After securing access with a 6F sheath, the latter would be removed on a 0.035-in wire placed into the ascending aortic root and exchanged for the sheathless 8F system, composed of a long 6F Shuttle Sheath (Cook) dilator inserted inside the 8F GC. Once the GC would reach the aorta, the dilator would be removed and the GC placed in the coronary.

However, 8F sheathless access has progressively become exceptional with the advent of thin-wall Slender Sheaths and miniaturization of microcatheters and the StingRay LP, alongside with the new TrapLiner. It now is used almost exclusively when an 8F GC is proved necessary over a 7F, like for ipsilateral retrograde approach using 1 GC.

Glidesheath Slender sheaths (Terumo, Shibuya-ku, Tokyo, Japan, and Merit Medical, South Jordan, UT, USA) have revolutionized the field of transradial complex PCI. They allow for the use of a 7F GC into a sheath that has the outer diameter of a 6F sheath, limiting trauma to the RA and expanding its use even in small women. With a 7F GC, the Stingray LP balloon can be used and trapped without friction.

The risk of RAO in regular PCI has been shown to be small and clinically insignificant (5.5% after 1 week of follow-up).[20] CTO PCI patients typically undergo several angiographies and PCIs prior to the CTO intervention. Therefore, the RA may not be available in some cases due to its occlusion. Use of higher dose of heparin (5000 units) and shorter compression times during these prior procedures may decrease its incidence.[20]

The RA offers less GC support, because most of the time it has to rely on active support, with minimal passive support. To mitigate this, the operator may choose to use guide-extensions and the crisscross technique (the GC coming from the right RA goes to the left coronary and

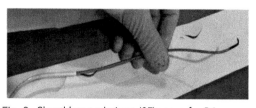

Fig. 3. Sheathless technique (8F) setup for RA access.

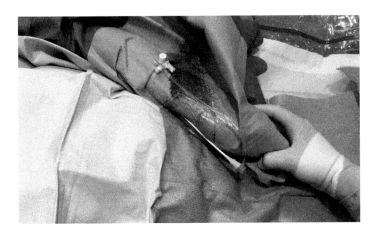

Fig. 4. Left distal radial access hack: use of a long 25 cm sheath keeping externalized (outside the body) approximately 10 cm of the sheath, taped on the hand, to easy manipulation and increase operator comfort.

the GC coming from the left RA goes to the right coronary artery). Using the left RA, however, may be uncomfortable for some operators (especially in obese patients). Novel developments, such as use of distal RA entry point, may ease that aspect. The authors propose an alternative approach, described as the left distal radial access hack, which consists of using a long 25 cm sheath and keeping externalized (outside the body) approximately 15 cm of the sheath, taped on the hand. This way, the hub of the sheath comes closer to the operator, easing manipulation (Fig. 4).

Patients with known occluded carotid or vertebral arteries, depending on collateral flow to the brain, may not be the ideal candidate for CTO PCI through the RA, having a catheter in front of the carotid or vertebral ostium for hours.

Finally, aorto-ostial CTOs, or CTOs with limited landing zone, are difficult to treat from the RA. The GC needs a good sitting and stable position in the coronary ostium for the RA to be effective, because the tip of the GC tends to disengage with breathing and lowering of the diaphragm with inspiration, which does not occur from the femoral (see Fig. 1).[6]

FEMORAL ARTERY AND RADIAL ARTERY TECHNIQUES
Radial Access
Access to the radial should be performed with a commercially available hydrophilic sheath, which reduces RAO. The authors favor the use of 6F to7F slender sheaths, especially if the radial is used for the antegrade GC. In cases of bilateral radial access, both can be done simultaneously (with an assistant) or sequentially. Use of long 25-cm sheaths avoids spasm with GC manipulation at the smaller segments of the artery and

allows for the sheath to be left out of the left RA, easing manipulations (Fig. 5).

To maintain the left arm in place, especially with obese patients, it is important to put the left wrist in supination, for comfort, and to tape the left elbow across the patient's chest up to the right side of the table for good support. The right arm also should be put in supination once the GCs have been positioned for shoulder comfort. The authors advocate the use of the left radial for the right coronary GC, and the right radial for the left coronary GC, irrespective of the location of the CTO. Therefore, the 7F antegrade GC is inserted through the left radial with an RCA CTO and through the right radial with a left-sided CTO. Although some new curves have been found helpful in

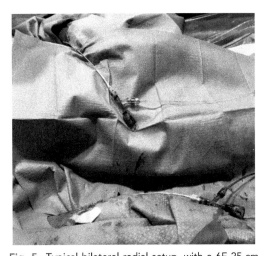

Fig. 5. Typical bilateral radial setup, with a 6F 25-cm sheath left 10 cm out of the left radial and a 6F guide to the right coronary artery (retrograde), and a 7F guide through a 6/7F Glidesheath Slender sheath (Terumo, Shibuya-ku, Tokyo, Japan) in the right radial to the left main coronary artery.

selective cases, use of extra back-up curves (XB or EBU) in the left main coronary artery and AL (Amplatz left) in the RCA are preferred, as from the FA. Although the authors recommend the use of the FA for SVGs, the left radial is well suited for SVGs to the RCA but provides limited support in an SVG to the left system.[21] In the latter situation, use of a guide-extension catheter often is extremely helpful. The RA also can be used for ipsilateral IMA cannulation; use of guide-extension catheters in such cases can be of great help. The authors strongly discourage the use of 5F GCs for CTO PCI, because it strongly limits options, unless a retrograde intervention is not foreseen and only contralateral injection is used.

As discussed previously, although the ulnar access has been used safely in non-CTO PCI, its safety in CTO PCI has not been studied extensively. The authors have used it a few occasions, with similar success and safety compared with the RA. The RA, however, should remain the default approach.

Femoral Access

State-of-the-art practice of FA has evolved from radiology-guided puncture using large-bore needles to ultrasound-guided puncture with microneedles.[22–24] The classic sweet spot of good femoral access, however, remains the same irrespective of technique; the common FA needs to be accessed above the bifurcation, to avoid superficial and/or profunda puncture and increase in the risk of pseudoaneurysm and hematoma, and low enough to avoid the risk of retroperitoneal bleed, below the inferior epigastric artery. It increasingly is recognized that the FA needs to be accessed over the superior pubic ramus, allowing for subsequent compression in case of bleeding.[24] Use of 45-cm sheath is advocated strongly, to improve support in all cases, easing manipulation of GCs through tortuous iliacs. Use of closure device is recommended in absence of contraindications.[24]

The FA remains the default access site for LV assist device. Proper techniques, including best access practices, use of preclosing, and close monitoring of anticoagulation with serial activated clotting time (ACT), is paramount to reduce the expected high rate of vascular and bleeding complications with these devices.

COMPLICATION MANAGEMENT

Local vascular complications at the site of catheter insertion constitute the most common adverse events after cardiovascular intervention, occurring in 1.4% of RA cases and 3.7% of FA cases (OR 0.37; 95% CI, 0.27–0.52; $P<.0001$).[8] Like in any other PCI, CTO PCI may lead to injury and vascular complications. Given the common use of dual access, and sometimes multiple accesses, it is reasonable to assume that this risk is higher in CTO PCI. Management of those complications, however, is similar to that of regular PCI.

The first step in complication management is to avoid it. Use of proper technique and equipment and adjunctive imaging (ultrasound, fluoroscopy, and occasionally computed tomography) are ways of making the procedure safer. Understanding the several factors and independent predictors associated with increased incidence of vascular complications also plays an important role (Box 1).[25–28]

Table 3 presents a list of complications, their incidences, and management according to the puncture site. The most common complications remain puncture site oozing, bruising, and hematoma.[29] Although hematomas per se have not been correlated with impaired long-term outcomes, they remain a significant source of morbidity and costs, often prolonging hospitalization.

Box 1
Factors associated with vascular complications

Nonmodifiable

1. Gender (women > men)
2. Age (older > younger)
3. Obesity
4. Peripheral vascular disease
5. Chronic kidney disease
6. Blood dyscrasia

Modifiable

1. Puncture site (CFA < SFA or EIA)
2. Sheath size (5F–6F <7F–8F)
3. Anticoagulation regimen (heparin bolus < heparin bolus + infusion, bivalirudin < heparin + GPI)
4. Puncture type (anterior wall < posterior wall, higher vs lower stick) (for FA)
5. FA + vein puncture (arteriovenous fistula)

Abbreviations: CFA, common FA; EIA, external iliac artery; GPI, glycoprotein inhibitor; SFA, superficial FA.

Table 3
Arterial access complications, incidence, and management

Complication	Incidence	Management
Hematoma (>5–10 cm)	Femoral: <5% Radial: 1%–3%	Management varies according to the size 1. Analgesia, additional compression, and local ice 2. Insufflate blood pressure cuff (if upper limb) 3. Surgery
Retroperitoneal bleeding	Femoral: <2% Radial: N/A	1. Early recognition (acquisition of a femoral angiogram may allow detection for active bleeding) 2. Computed tomography imaging with contrast 3. Surgery
Pseudoaneurysm	Femoral: <1%–2% Radial: <0.1%	1. Echo-guided compression 2. Thrombin injection 3. Surgery
Arteriovenous fistula	Femoral: <1%–2% Radial: <0.1%	1. Conservative management (most will have spontaneous resolution) 2. Surgery
Thrombosis/embolism (limb ischemia)	Femoral: <0.1% Radial: 0.8%–10% at hospital discharge (limb ischemia extremely rare)	1. Endovascular or open surgery repair
Infection	Femoral: <5% Radial: <0.1%	1. Any persistent discomfort over the arterial puncture should prompt investigation to exclude vascular complications and local sepsis, especially if vascular closure devices were used
Dissection/perforation	Femoral: <1% Radial: <1%	1. Conservative management (blood flow will facilitate adherence of vessel layers and promote healing) 2. An alternative access may be needed 3. Endovascular repair 4. Surgery (especially in compartment syndrome)
Compartment syndrome	Femoral: very rare Radial: <0.01%	1. Stop intravenous anticoagulant therapy 2. Pain and blood pressure control 3. Use of transient external compression (with blood pressure cuff if upper limb) 4. Open surgical fasciotomy

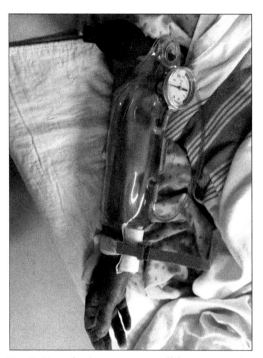

Fig. 6. Use of a bag pressure cuff for compression: avoiding compartment syndrome of the forearm after arterial perforation.

Early recognition of a vascular complication facilitates its management. Most of the complications can be dealt with conservative management. Up to 5% of the FA and 0.1% of the RA vascular complications, however, need surgical repair.[25,27]

The small diameter of the RA combined with its superficial location makes the incidence of vascular complications limited compared with the FA, and, more importantly, clinical consequences are relatively more benign. The downside of the smaller and muscular RA is its propensity to spasm or occlusion. The incidence of RA spasm is approximately 30% to 35%, but it

can be strongly dramatically reduced to less than 15% with the use of prophylactic cocktails.[30] The optimal pharmacologic agent or combination of agents remains to be determined. In cases of severe spasm, papaverine, profound analgesia, or local anesthesia may be required. Rare cases of partial or complete RA avulsion have been described and require surgery.[31] RAO is a common complication after RA access and found more common in women, the elderly, and patients with diabetes, smaller radial size, larger sheath size, and low or no heparin dosage. Strategies to avoid RAO have been developed and can reduce the incidence to below 2%. RAOs, however, almost invariably are asymptomatic and only preclude the use of this access site in future catheterizations; as such, use of a larger GC through the RA, which may lead to its subsequent thrombotic occlusion, should be put into perspective to the prevention of potentially more serious femoral complications.

Vessel perforation and dissection may occur throughout the arterial path when the RA is used due to anatomic variations, severe tortuosity, or loops. These complications can be sealed once the GC carefully is crossed over a 0.014-in guide wire, with no clinical consequence for the patient. Failure to recognize these perforations, however, might be dramatic because slow and delayed intramuscular bleeding potentially may lead to compartment syndrome.

Although RAO usually is benign clinically, an RA perforation can lead to rare but dramatic complications, such as compartment syndrome and need for fasciotomy. RA perforation often occurs from catheter exchanges, with razor-edge effect that may traumatize the main vessel or its side branches. To avoid compartment syndrome, early recognition of forearm hematoma should trigger fast and protocolized management with external compression of the perforation site. A blood pressure cuff, or

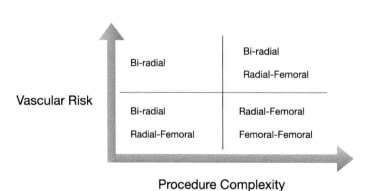

Fig. 7. Selection of arterial access for CTO PCI according to procedure complexity and vascular risk.

more practically a bag pressure cuff (Fig. 6), blown to a pressure that leads to loss of distal capillary pulse wave and then released slowly to allow pulsatility to come back, can be used for compression. The cuff is locked at this pressure for 2 hours and usually stops externalization of blood from the artery.

Some types of vascular closure devices have been associated with reports of FA thrombosis or limb ischemia due to embolization of foreign material or in situ thrombus formation on the intravascular device components. Infection, although described without the use of vascular closure devices (0.6%), has been associated with different vascular closure devices.[32]

Finally, although very high level of anticoagulation may be less consequential with the RA, very high ACTs should be avoided when an FA is used.

SUMMARY

Both accesses have important advantages and disadvantages. The FA has more procedural advantages with some important disadvantages in terms of harder outcomes. The RA is safer but may create some procedural challenges in some determined cases. Determining the ratio risk/benefit–efficacy/safety of each access for each patient in a specific procedure should be based on coronary anatomy, clinical characteristics, vascular access difficulties, and potential strategies and devices that are used.

Overall, given the safety benefit and the minimal procedural disadvantages with the technologies and strategies current available, the authors advocate use of at least 1 RA, ideally dual RA accesses, as the standard approach in most cases, especially in procedures of low complexity and in patients at high risk of vascular complications (Fig. 7). Nonetheless, it is imperative that CTO operators master both approaches because they are needed in multiple occasions, such as in post-CABG patients (with the use of triple access for adequate visualization of the target vessel), in high-risk patients (with the use of mechanical circulatory support), and in patients with multiple prior angiographies (who may have RAO or severe fibrosis at the puncture site).

CLINICAL CARE POINTS

- Bilateral radial approach should be used when possible.

- GCs 6F usually are large enough for retrograde maneuvers.
- GCs 7F or 8F are very useful for antegrade techniques.
- Combined femoral and radial approaches increasingly are used to avoid the risk of bilateral femoral approach.
- Slender 6F to 7F guides have revolutionized complex PCI from the RA.
- New tools and techniques are available to ease the procedure.
- The femoral approach using a larger guide size provides better support and is mandatory when the landing zone of the guide is short or absent.

DISCLOSURE

The authors have nothing to disclose.

REFERENCES

1. Megaly M, Karatasakis A, Abraham B, et al. Radial versus femoral access in chronic total occlusion percutaneous coronary intervention. Circ Cardiovasc Interv 2019;12(6):e007778.
2. Tanaka Y, Moriyama N, Ochiai T, et al. Transradial coronary interventions for complex chronic total occlusions. JACC Cardiovasc Interv 2017;10(3): 235–43.
3. Tajti P, Alaswad K, Karmpaliotis D, et al. Procedural Outcomes of Percutaneous Coronary Interventions for Chronic Total Occlusions Via the Radial Approach: Insights From an International Chronic Total Occlusion Registry. JACC Cardiovasc Interv 2019;12(4):346–58.
4. Burzotta F, De Vita M, Lefevre T, et al. Radial approach for percutaneous coronary interventions on chronic total occlusions: technical issues and data review. Catheter Cardiovasc Interv 2014; 83(1):47–57.
5. Kinnaird T, Anderson R, Ossei-Gerning N, et al. Vascular Access Site and Outcomes Among 26,807 Chronic Total Coronary Occlusion Angioplasty Cases From the British Cardiovascular Interventions Society National Database. JACC Cardiovasc Interv 2017;10(7):635–44.
6. Rinfret S, Dautov R. Radial or Femoral Approach for Chronic Total Occlusion Revascularization?: The Answer Is Both. JACC Cardiovasc Interv 2017; 10(3):244–6.
7. Fairley SL, Lucking AJ, McEntegart M, et al. Routine Use of Fluoroscopic-Guided Femoral Arterial Puncture to Minimise Vascular Complication Rates in CTO Intervention: Multi-centre UK Experience. Heart Lung Circ 2016;25(12):1203–9.

8. Jolly SS, Yusuf S, Cairns J, et al. Radial versus femoral access for coronary angiography and intervention in patients with acute coronary syndromes (RIVAL): a randomised, parallel group, multicentre trial. Lancet 2011;377(9775):1409–20.

9. Romagnoli E, Biondi-Zoccai G, Sciahbasi A, et al. Radial versus femoral randomized investigation in ST-segment elevation acute coronary syndrome: the RIFLE-STEACS (Radial Versus Femoral Randomized Investigation in ST-Elevation Acute Coronary Syndrome) study. J Am Coll Cardiol 2012; 60(24):2481–9.

10. Bernat I, Horak D, Stasek J, et al. ST-segment elevation myocardial infarction treated by radial or femoral approach in a multicenter randomized clinical trial: the STEMI-RADIAL trial. J Am Coll Cardiol 2014;63(10):964–72.

11. Ferrante G, Rao SV, Juni P, et al. Radial Versus Femoral Access for Coronary Interventions Across the Entire Spectrum of Patients With Coronary Artery Disease: A Meta-Analysis of Randomized Trials. JACC Cardiovasc Interv 2016;9(14):1419–34.

12. Bagur R, Rinfret S. Transradial Approach for Chronic Total Occlusion Percutaneous Coronary Intervention. Interv Cardiol Clin 2012;1(3):355–63.

13. Fernandez R, Zaky F, Ekmejian A, et al. Safety and efficacy of ulnar artery approach for percutaneous cardiac catheterization: Systematic review and meta-analysis. Catheter Cardiovasc Interv 2018; 91(7):1273–80.

14. Kedev S, Zafirovska B, Dharma S, et al. Safety and feasibility of transulnar catheterization when ipsilateral radial access is not available. Catheter Cardiovasc Interv 2014;83(1):E51–60.

15. Koutouzis M, Ziakas A, Didagelos M, et al. Ipsilateral radial and ulnar artery cannulation during the same coronary catheterization procedure. Hippokratia 2016;20(3):249–51.

16. Mason PJ, Shah B, Tamis-Holland JE, et al. An Update on Radial Artery Access and Best Practices for Transradial Coronary Angiography and Intervention in Acute Coronary Syndrome: A Scientific Statement From the American Heart Association. Circ Cardiovasc Interv 2018;11(9):e000035.

17. Rinfret S, Joyal D, Nguyen CM, et al. Retrograde recanalization of chronic total occlusions from the transradial approach; early Canadian experience. Catheter Cardiovasc Interv 2011;78(3):366–74.

18. Azzalini L, Dautov R, Brilakis ES, et al. Procedural and longer-term outcomes of wire- versus device-based antegrade dissection and re-entry techniques for the percutaneous revascularization of coronary chronic total occlusions. Int J Cardiol 2017;231:78–83.

19. Dautov R, Ribeiro HB, Abdul-Jawad Altisent O, et al. Effectiveness and Safety of the Transradial 8Fr Sheathless Approach for Revascularization of Chronic Total Occlusions. Am J Cardiol 2016; 118(6):785–9.

20. Rashid M, Kwok CS, Pancholy S, et al. Radial Artery Occlusion After Transradial Interventions: A Systematic Review and Meta-Analysis. J Am Heart Assoc 2016;5(1):e002686.

21. Israeli Z, Lavi S, Pancholy SB, et al. Radial versus femoral approach for saphenous vein grafts angiography and interventions. Am Heart J 2019;210:1–8.

22. Ben-Dor I, Maluenda G, Mahmoudi M, et al. A novel, minimally invasive access technique versus standard 18-gauge needle set for femoral access. Catheter Cardiovasc Interv 2012;79(7):1180–5.

23. Seto AH, Abu-Fadel MS, Sparling JM, et al. Real-time ultrasound guidance facilitates femoral arterial access and reduces vascular complications: FAUST (Femoral Arterial Access With Ultrasound Trial). JACC Cardiovasc Interv 2010;3(7):751–8.

24. Sandoval Y, Burke MN, Lobo AS, et al. Contemporary Arterial Access in the Cardiac Catheterization Laboratory. JACC Cardiovasc Interv 2017;10(22): 2233–41.

25. Chandrasekar B, Doucet S, Bilodeau L, et al. Complications of cardiac catheterization in the current era: a single-center experience. Catheter Cardiovasc Interv 2001;52(3):289–95.

26. Sherev DA, Shaw RE, Brent BN. Angiographic predictors of femoral access site complications: implication for planned percutaneous coronary intervention. Catheter Cardiovasc Interv 2005; 65(2):196–202.

27. Kanei Y, Kwan T, Nakra NC, et al. Transradial cardiac catheterization: a review of access site complications. Catheter Cardiovasc Interv 2011;78(6):840–6.

28. Grossman PM, Gurm HS, McNamara R, et al. Percutaneous coronary intervention complications and guide catheter size: bigger is not better. JACC Cardiovasc Interv 2009;2(7):636–44.

29. Cosman TL, Arthur HM, Natarajan MK. Prevalence of bruising at the vascular access site one week after elective cardiac catheterisation or percutaneous coronary intervention. J Clin Nurs 2011;20(9–10): 1349–56.

30. Kiemeneij F, Vajifdar BU, Eccleshall SC, et al. Evaluation of a spasmolytic cocktail to prevent radial artery spasm during coronary procedures. Catheter Cardiovasc Interv 2003;58(3):281–4.

31. Dieter RS, Akef A, Wolff M. Eversion endarterectomy complicating radial artery access for left heart catheterization. Catheter Cardiovasc Interv 2003; 58(4):478–80.

32. Nikolsky E, Mehran R, Halkin A, et al. Vascular complications associated with arteriotomy closure devices in patients undergoing percutaneous coronary procedures: a meta-analysis. J Am Coll Cardiol 2004;44(6):1200–9.

Patient and Device Selection for Hemodynamic Support in High-Risk Percutaneous Coronary Intervention

Rhian E. Davies, DO, MS[a,1,*], Jeremy D. Rier, DO[a,1], James M. McCabe, MD[b]

KEYWORDS

- Mechanical circulatory support • High-risk PCI • Large bore • Access

---

KEY POINTS

- The term and concepts surrounding high-risk percutaneous coronary intervention (PCI) include many patient subsets, such as multivessel coronary artery disease, intervention of the last remaining vessel, a severely stenotic unprotected left main (particularly in a left dominant coronary artery circulation), acute myocardial infarction complicated by cardiogenic shock, and depressed left ventricular ejection fraction.
- Mechanical circulatory support may help overcome hemodynamic, ischemic, and arrhythmic challenges during high-risk PCI.
- Interventionalists should be familiar with the advantages, disadvantages, and when value is added by the use of both right-sided and left-sided mechanical circulatory support devices.

INTRODUCTION

The prevalence of high-risk coronary artery disease presenting to the cardiac catheterization laboratory has grown in recent decades, likely from increasing comorbidities, including diabetes, hypercholesterolemia, frailty, decreased left ventricular (LV) ejection fraction, and increasing age, along with consideration of patients turned down for surgical revascularization.[1-3] This has resulted in the evolution of percutaneous coronary techniques and subsequently the expansion of hemodynamic support options. The term, *high-risk percutaneous coronary intervention (PCI)*, remains poorly defined[4] but includes patients with multivessel coronary

artery disease, intervention of the last remaining vessel, and a severely stenotic unprotected left main coronary artery, particularly with left dominant circulation.[1-3] Additional considerations include acute myocardial infarction (MI) complicated with hemodynamic instability, significant arrythmias, acute decompensated heart failure, and those patients with limited improvement on vasopressors or inotropes and evidence of end-organ damage (such as elevated creatinine, lactate, troponin, and transaminitis).[1-3]

Patients undergoing high-risk procedures can develop hemodynamic instability, arrythmias, or even cardiac arrest as a result of ischemia, which can be brought on during use of specialized techniques, including atherectomy, retrograde

---

[a] Department of Cardiology, University of Washington Medical Center, Seattle, WA, USA; [b] Department of Cardiology, University of Washington Medical Center, 1959 Northeast Pacific Street Box 356422, Seattle, WA 98185, USA
[1] Present address: 1001 S George Street, York, PA 17403.
* Corresponding author.
E-mail address: rhian.elizabeth.davies@gmail.com
Twitter: @RhianEDavies1 (R.E.D.); @jeremyrier (J.D.R.); @J_M_McCabe (J.M.M.)

Intervent Cardiol Clin 10 (2021) 121–130
https://doi.org/10.1016/j.iccl.2020.09.001

chronic total occlusion PCI, or microvascular disruption from atheroembolic debris. Therefore, having the proficiency to insert and manage percutaneous mechanical circulatory support (MCS) devices can be advantageous in maintaining or even improving coronary perfusion pressure during critical times. In addition, these devices can reduce the myocardial workload in the periprocedure time frame, potentially allowing patients to have improved outcomes. Algorithms can help guide decision making when considering MCS for high-risk PCI (Fig. 1). This proposed algorithm requires evaluation of hemodynamics, clinical presentation, and procedural factors that would increase the risk of the procedure. A point system is allocated for each factor. Patients with 0 to 2 points are unlikely to need support whereas support should be considered when patients have 3 points. Furthermore, if a patient has 4 or more points, support should be strongly considered.[5] Although multiple algorithms for patient selection of MCS exist, ongoing research will help identify clinical scenarios and patients who benefit most from its use. The ideal MCS device would include a straightforward insertion without the need for surgical vascular access, easy initiation, and subsequent maintenance of the device and have the ability to provide durable perfusion of the peripheral and coronary circulation for hours to days.[6] This article discusses the options for both left-sided and right-sided MCS devices for which highlights are provided in Tables 1 and 2.

LEFT-SIDED MECHANICAL CIRCULATORY SUPPORT
Intra-aortic Balloon Pump
The intra-aortic balloon pump (IABP) is a readily available support device found in the majority of cardiac catheterization laboratories. The IABP first was used in 1968 for a patient with cardiogenic shock secondary to an acute MI.[7] It was further validated to improve cardiac output (CO) in a study conducted by Jacobey,[8] who investigated its use in 18 patients with cardiogenic shock. It requires a 7 French (F), 7.5F, or 8F access and typically is inserted into either the femoral or axillary arteries. The IABP provides an internal counterpulsation, which improves circulation as a result of diastolic augmentation.[7] It inflates during diastole and deflates during systole. Although the device inflates, it increases blood flow to the coronary, cerebral, and systemic circulation.[7] Theoretically, as a result of the timing of inflation and deflation, it can decrease the myocardial work and oxygen demand while increasing the CO by 0.5 L to 1 L per minute.

The timing of inflation and deflation of the IABP can occur in conjunction with the electrocardiogram timing or pressure changes. The balloon inflates at the initiation of diastole and deflate in systole. The inflation can give rise to improved myocardial perfusion by increasing the coronary pressure gradient from the aorta to the epicardial coronary circulation. When the balloon inflates, there is a displacement of blood, which results in redistribution of blood flow and alteration of oxygen consumption.[9,10] The magnitude of the effect of balloon inflation and deflation relies on its size in proportion to the aorta.[6] The larger the balloon, the more volume of blood displaced; therefore, the maximal size appropriate for the patient is important. Ideally, the balloon should extend distal to the take-off of the left subclavian and end short of the take-off of the celiac artery. This prevents any unwanted complications, including intermittent occlusion

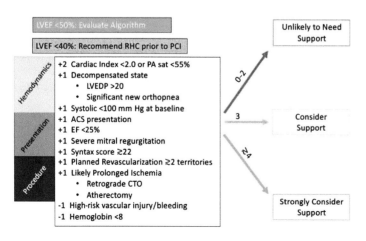

Fig. 1. Suggested patient selection algorithm for MCS use in high-risk PCI. BP, blood pressure; CTO, chronic total occlusion; EF, ejection fraction; LVEDP; LV end-diastolic pressure; PA sat, PA saturation; PCI, percutaneous coronary intervention; RHC, right heart catheterization.

Table 1			
Advantages and disadvantages of the available left-sided mechanical circulatory support devices for high-risk percutaneous coronary intervention			
Mechanical Circulatory Support Device	Features: • Augmentation of Cardiac Output • Sheath Size • Access Routes	Advantages	Disadvantages
IABP	• 0.3–1 L/min • 7F, 7.5F, 8F • Femoral or axillary artery	• Available in most cardiac catheterization laboratories • Easy to insert • Automatic calibration • Range of balloon sizes	• Requires native CO • Not reliable if in unstable rhythm • Risk of balloon twisting or kinking resulting in rupture or leakage of internal helium. • Aortic damage if preexisting aortic disorder or using too large of a balloon
Impella	• 2.5 L/min or 4 L/min (Impella CP) • 12F–14F • Femoral or axillary	• Can be used for an extended duration (7 or more days) • Does not rely on stable rhythm or native CO	• Requires adequate LV filling • Not universally available • Can be inadvertently displaced from the LV • Contraindicated with LV thrombus, mechanical aortic valve, severe AI • Large-bore arterial access may cause ischemia requiring reperfusion sheath placement • Risk of hemolysis • Risk of vascular and bleeding complications
TH	• 4–5 L/min • 21F venous and 15F–17F arterial sheaths • Femoral artery and vein	• Can be used for extended duration (14 or more days) • Does not rely on stable rhythm or native CO • Can be used if a patient has an LV thrombus or a mechanical aortic valve	• Not universally available • Requires transseptal puncture; preferred TEE or ICE guidance • Can be removed inadvertently from the LA, resulting in profound desaturation and patient instability • Large-bore arterial access may cause ischemia requiring reperfusion sheath placement • Risk of hemolysis • Risk of vascular and bleeding complications

(continued on next page)

VA-ECMO	• 4.5 L/min • 17F–19F for arterial and 21F–24F for venous sheaths • Femoral artery and vein (alternative access sites if obtained by cardiothoracic surgery)	• Can be used for extended duration (several weeks) • Does not rely on stable rhythm or native CO	• Limited by resource utilization (center dependent) • Lung injury may occur • Poor coronary and cerebral perfusion • Increased myocardial workload, therefore may require venting/unloading of the LV • Large-bore arterial access may cause ischemia requiring reperfusion sheath placement • Risk of hemolysis • Risk of vascular and bleeding complications

of the renal arteries. The balloon does come in a variety of sizes, including 25 cm^3, 30 cm^3, 34 cm^3, 40 cm^3, and 50 cm^3. The 40-cm^3 size likely is the most commonly used in an adult. It is important to realize that if too large an IABP is placed, there is a heightened risk of vascular morbidity, whereas if too small an IABP is placed, there would a reduction in the cardiac benefits.[7]

Additionally, if a patient has an increased heart rate, therefore decreasing the duration of diastole, or has a low systemic vascular resistance, the IABP does not provide the same effect. Data regarding the use and outcomes of IABP over the past several decades have demonstrated a decrease of in-hospital mortality and lower catheterization laboratory-related events. Unfortunately, this is conflicted by many studies showing no benefit with the use of the IABP and even a trend toward harm.[2,6,11–16]

Percutaneous, Left-Sided Transvalvular Heart Pumps

The currently available coaxial, transvalvular devices for ventricular unloading are the Impella family of devices (Abiomed, Danvers, Massachusetts), which increasingly are used for high-risk PCI.[17] The Impella 2.5 and Impella CP are advanced percutaneously in a retrograde

Table 2
Advantages and disadvantages of the available right-sided mechanical circulatory support devices for high-risk percutaneous coronary intervention

Mechanical Circulatory Support Device	Features: • Flow • Sheath Size • Access Routes	Advantages	Disadvantages
Impella RP	• ~3 L/min • 22F • Right femoral vein (preferred)	• Decrease in RA pressure • Increase in cardiac index • Decreased need for inotropic support	• Unable to ambulate • Large-bore access increasing risk of bleeding or vascular complications
ProtekDuo	• 4.5–5 L/min • 29F • Right internal jugular vein (preferred) or subclavian vein	• Decrease in RA pressure • Increase in cardiac index • Decreased need for inotropic support • Able to ambulate	• Large-bore access increasing risk of bleeding or vascular complications

fashion across the aortic valve into the LV via the femoral or axillary artery. This group of devices have a miniaturized rotary pump, allowing blood to be pulled from the LV and displaced into the ascending aorta. These devices may decrease end diastolic wall stress, thus improving diastolic compliance and ultimately allowing a decrease in coronary microvascular resistance as a result of increasing aortic and intracoronary pressure.[18,19] The Impella 2.5 delivers up to 2.5 L/min and the Impella CP delivers up to 4 L/min. Additional Impella devices include the Impella 5.0 and Impella LD, which require surgical assistance for placement, although more recently, transcaval techniques have been utilized for fully percutaneous Impella 5.0 insertion.[20]

In the Prospective Feasibility Trial Investigating the Use of IMPELLA RECOVER LP 2.5 System in Patients Undergoing High-Risk PCI (PROTECT I) trial, the Impella 2.5 was investigated for hemodynamic support during high-risk PCI and demonstrated adequate safe and facile insertion in this early experience.[1] In the Prospective Randomized Clinical Trial of Hemodynamic Support with Impella 2.5 versus Intra-Aortic Balloon Pump in Patients Undergoing High-Risk PCI (PROTECT II) trial, high-risk PCI was considered unprotected left main or last patent conduit and an LV ejection fraction less than or equal to 35% or with 3-vessel disease and an LV ejection fraction less than or equal to 30%. Although negative for the primary outcome at 30 days, the 90-day outcomes, which included intraprocedural and postprocedural major adverse events, demonstrated that use of Impella 2.5 resulted in improved outcomes in comparison to IABP in per protocol analysis.[21]

Because this device requires advancement across the aortic valve, the operator needs to understand that severe or critical aortic stenosis may make the delivery of this device difficult, especially in urgent scenarios. The IABP and Impella devices are contraindicated in cases of significant aortic regurgitation. Additionally, the operator should rule out concerns for possible LV thrombus for those individuals with a reduced LV ejection fraction for a prolonged duration who are not on anticoagulation, especially in cases of apical infarct. Other concerns with the Impella involve concern for hemolysis and access site complications, including bleeding and ischemia.[17] The Impella 2.5 requires a 13F sheath and the Impella CP requires a 14F sheath.

TandemHeart

The TandemHeart (TH) ventricular assist device (LivaNova, London, United Kingdom) is a centrifugal pump that also functions to unload the LV but in a different method. A 21F venous cannula is advanced via the femoral vein to the right atrium (RA) and ultimately into the left atrium via a transseptal puncture. A second 15F to 17F cannula, which acts as an outflow tract, is inserted into the femoral artery extending to the aortic bifurcation. Therefore, this device provides a partial cardiac bypass circuit at flow rate of 4 L/min.

Use of a transesophageal echocardiogram (TEE) is recommended for placement of the TH device. The fossa ovalis can be visualized in the midesophageal bicaval view, which is the thinnest portion of the intra-atrial septum and the ideal location for trans-septal puncture. A midesophageal short axis view of the aortic valve can be obtained (typically at 40°–50°) to avoid inadvertent puncture of the aorta or atrial wall. Intracardiac echocardiogram (ICE) is an alternative to aid fluoroscopic placement during transseptal puncture.

The TH compared with the Impella 2.5 demonstrated equal effectiveness and was associated with similar short-term and long-term clinical outcomes for 68 patients undergoing high-risk PCI in a study by Kovacic and colleagues[22] In this study, 32 patients received a TH and 36 received an Impella 2.5.[22] They had a 99% PCI success rate in both groups with similar in-hospital outcomes and a combined 7% major vascular access site complication rate. The 30-day MACE rate (death, MI, and target lesion revascularization) was 5.8%.[22] Additional observational studies have demonstrated that the TH allows for reduction of the pulmonary capillary wedge pressure and pulmonary artery (PA) and central venous pressures, resulting in decreased filling pressures and ultimately a decrease in myocardial workload.[23–25]

Extracorporeal Membrane Oxygenation

Venoarterial (VA)-extracorporeal membrane oxygenation (ECMO) is a modified cardiopulmonary bypass device that is able to provide patients with biventricular hemodynamic support and oxygenation via a continuous, nonpulsatile CO. There are 2 large-bore cannulas used in percutaneous peripheral VA-ECMO cannulation, one of which is advanced via a large vein with destination in the RA and the other is advanced via a large artery with destination in the aorta. This device functions to provide circulatory support while removing deoxygenated blood through a membrane which is external to the body and replacing it with oxygenated blood.

In a retrospective analysis comparing prophylactic VA-ECMO to standby VA-ECMO for patients undergoing high-risk PCI, there was a significant increase in procedural morbidity from femoral access site complications in the prophylactic cohort (41% vs 9.4%. respectively; $P<.01$). The standby cohort, however, had a higher procedural mortality (4.8% vs 18.8%, respectively; $P<.05$).[26] Therefore, from this study, it is suggested that patients with an EF of less than 20% may benefit from standby VA-ECMO compared with prophylactic VA-ECMO secondary to the increased risk of vascular complications.[26] Patients presenting with ST-elevation MI and cardiogenic shock undergoing primary PCI were found to have a reduction in 30-day mortality when they received early placement of VA-ECMO compared with patients who did not receive support.[27]

Aside from vascular access complications, VA-ECMO subjects the patient to complications similar to the Impella and TH support devices, including hemolysis, limb ischemia, and coagulation concerns. Importantly, VA-ECMO has been shown to increase LV afterload and wall stress. This subsequently results in an increase in myocardial oxygen consumption leading to an increase in myocardial infarct size.[28] Ultimately, this may prevent recovery of the myocardium; therefore, venting or unloading the LV should be considered (IABP, percutaneous ventricular assist device, or pulmonary vein or transseptal left atrial cannulation) in the ischemic patient. Other concerns with this device include patients with peripheral vascular disease and patients with bleeding issues as this device requires large-bore access and anticoagulation when in use.[29]

RIGHT-SIDED MECHANICAL CIRCULATORY SUPPORT

Many patients who present with right coronary artery infarcts may go on to develop right-sided heart failure. Occasionally, these patients may require MCS when inotropes and vasopressors simply are not enough. Additionally, patients who receive left-sided MCS may develop decompensation of their right ventricle (RV), creating another situation whereby right-sided MCS would be indicated.

In determining if RV MCS support is necessary, an operator can calculate a PA pulsatility index (PI), also known as a PAPi score.[30] This is the difference between PA systolic and diastolic pressure divided by their RA pressure.[30] If this value is noted to be less than 0.9 in the setting of acute coronary syndrome (ACS), the RV is considered dysfunctional, although a PAPi less than 1.85 has been associated with RV failure after continuous-flow LV assist device (LVAD) surgery in a single-center study.[31]

The RV pushes blood into the pulmonary system, which, by nature, is a compliant low-resistance area; therefore, the RV systolic pressure does not need to be very high to work effectively. When patients have ischemia of their RV, however, such as with ACS, the end-diastolic volume increases and, because the RV is sensitive to loading conditions, failure may quickly ensue.[32,33] This may result in a decrease in CO with subsequent reduction in systemic perfusion causing a neurohormonal response with cytokine release and mechanical-stretch signaling, ultimately causing necrosis and cell death.[32,33] In many cases of biventricular or right-sided failure, ECMO may be selected up front, but in several situations, where LVAD support is insufficient or with isolated RV failure, a right-sided devices is considered. Therefore, it is important to realize the advantages and disadvantages of the 2 currently available options for percutaneous right-sided mechanical support.

Impella RP

The Impella RP is an axial flow pump with a 22F pump motor that is advanced via the right femoral vein into the RA across the tricuspid and pulmonic valves, with its ultimate destination within the left (preferred) or right PA. The inlet, therefore, is located within the inferior vena cava and the outflow is located in the PA.[34] As a result of entry location, the patient must remain on bedrest while this device remains in place. In the Impella RP trial, patients with RV failure (after LVAD or postcardiotomy) had an average flow of 3 L/min, with improvements in RA pressures, cardiac index, and decreased need for inotropic support.[35]

In a retrospective study of 18 patients, after placement of this device, they were noted to have an increase in cardiac index (2.1 L/min/m^2 $\pm$ 0.1 L/min/m^2 preimplant vs 2.6 L/min/m^2 $\pm$ 0.2 L/min/m^2 postimplant; $P = .04$) and a reduction of central venous pressure (22 mm Hg $\pm$ 5 mm Hg vs 15 mm Hg $\pm$ 4 mm Hg; $P<.01$).[36] Additionally, in the RECOVER RIGHT study, 30 patients were evaluated with RV failure refractory to medical treatment received the Impella RP device. Of the 30, there were 18 patients with RV failure after LVAD implantation (cohort A) and 12 patients with RV failure after cardiotomy or MI (cohort B).[37] Immediately after insertion, there was improvement seen in hemodynamics, with an increase in cardiac index from 1.8 L/min/m^2 ± 0.2 L/min/m^2 to 3.3 L/min/m^2 ± 0.23 L/min/m^2 (P<.001) and a decrease in central venous pressure from 19.2 mm Hg ± 4 mm Hg to 12.6 mm Hg ± 1 mm Hg (P<.001).[37] Real-world experience has been limited in the critically ill patients, possibly due to late recognition, but have given pause to broader adoption and emphasize the importance of patient selection.[38]

ProtekDuo

The ProtekDuo (LivaNova) is a 29F dual-lumen cannula that can be inserted percutaneously via either the internal jugular or subclavian veins to the RA, past the tricuspid valve through the RV, and eventually out past the pulmonic valve into the main PA. The proximal inflow lumen is positioned in the RA and the distal outflow lumen is positioned in the main PA. Externally, the dual-lumen catheter is connected with the paracorporeal TH pump, allowing flows up to 4.5 L/min to 5 L/min[39] An oxygenator also can be introduced into the circuit if needed and available to allow full RV and oxygenation support.

In a retrospective study, where 13 patients received the ProtekDuo, only 4 patients suffered an acute MI complicated by cardiogenic shock and RV failure. Of these, 2 recovered to device explantation, where an additional 5 patients who also recovered had this device placed for various reasons, including post-LVAD implantation, bridge to heart or lung transplant, and acute myocarditis.[39]

An additional retrospective study that included 17 patients between 2 centers noted the ease of placement of the ProtekDuo and patients were able to gain support without the need of a sternotomy.[40] Unfortunately, mortality remained 40%,[40] emphasizing the poor outcomes associated with RV failure in cardiogenic shock.[41,42]

DISCUSSION

In total, data regarding device selection are confounded by selection bias and available trials limited in generalizability to the patients evaluated on a daily basis. A thorough assessment of the potential risks and benefits of intervention as well as MCS is paramount to case planning for high-risk PCI. A variety of clinical situations may place the patient at high risk for PCI due to patient reserve and are overlayed with technical factors relating to the likelihood of high ischemic burden and complication possibilities. Traditionally, depressed LV function, challenging coronary anatomy, last remaining conduit, and unprotected left main have been regarded as high risk, but patients with higher acuity due to decompensated heart failure, ACS presentations, or frank cardiogenic shock are emerging as the more pressing population requiring MCS during PCI. With advancing patient age, there is a heightened risk of mortality, bleeding, and vascular complications in dealing with large-bore catheters.[43–45] Comfort with access and managing its complications is a prerequisite for the high-risk PCI operator. Selected patients may not achieve adequate and successful revascularization without the use of a MCS devices and, therefore, potential benefit must be balanced with these real procedural risks.

As is known, if patients suffer from an acute MI and go on to develop cardiogenic shock, their rate of mortality is as high as 40% to 50%.[46,47] MCS, in particular, Impella and TH devices, have shown favorable changes in hemodynamic assessments by an improvement in cardiac index (CI), mean arterial pressure, and pulmonary capillary wedge pressure compared with the IABP in a meta-analysis conducted by Cheng and colleagues. Despite having to use a larger sheath size for both the Impella and TH, there was no significant difference observed in incidence of leg ischemia compared with IABP patients, although bleeding rates are observed to be higher.[48]

MCS devices can be necessary to overcome hemodynamic, ischemic, and arrhythmic challenges during a high-risk PCI. Knowledge not only of the indications but also of the contraindications, limitations, and availability of these devices is important for guiding device and patient selection. Additionally, if an MCS device is unable to be immediately removed post-PCI, multidisciplinary teams, including the proceduralist and critical care practitioners, are crucial for successful management. It also is essential to recognize the concerns that temper enthusiasm, despite their benefit during PCI; choose devices only when appropriate; and use best practices during device insertion and explantation.

CLINICS CARE POINTS

- Although not prospectively powered for the outcome, elective IABP use during PCI was associated with a 34% relative reduction in all-cause mortality compared with unsupported PCI.

- In as treated analysis, the use of Impella instead of IABP demonstrated a statistically significant reduction in major adverse events at 90 days.
- Use of Tandem Heart LV MCS may be useful in the presence of LV thrombus or a mechanical aortic valve.
- Use of the PAPi score can help guide the use of RV MCS.
- When using ECMO, LV venting/unloading may be helpful to reduce the myocardial work load and improve the likelihood of myocardial recovery.
- Data regarding device selection are confounded by selection bias and available trials limited in generalizability to the patients evaluated on a daily basis.

DISCLOSURE

Dr McCabe reports that CSI, Teleflex, Bos Sci are relevant conflicts. The other authors have nothing to disclose.

REFERENCES

1. Dixon SR, Henriques JPS, Mauri L, et al. A prospective feasibility trial investigating the use of the impella 2.5 system in patients undergoing high-risk percutaneous coronary intervention (The PROTECT I Trial). Initial U.S. experience. JACC Cardiovasc Interv 2009;2(2):91–6.
2. Mishra S, Chu WW, Torguson R, et al. Role of prophylactic intra-aortic balloon pump in high-risk patients undergoing percutaneous coronary intervention. Am J Cardiol 2006;98(5):608–12.
3. Dangas GD, Kini AS, Sharma SK, et al. Impact of hemodynamic support with impella 2.5 versus intra-aortic balloon pump on prognostically important clinical outcomes in patients undergoing high-risk percutaneous coronary intervention (from the PROTECT II Randomized Trial). Am J Cardiol 2014;113:222–8.
4. Kirtane AJ, Doshi D, Leon MB, et al. Treatment of higher-risk patients with an indication for revascularization. Circulation 2016;134(5):422–31.
5. Kearney KE, Mccabe JM, Riley RF. Patient selection and procedural strategy are key in treating this evolving patient population. Hemodynamic Support for High-Risk PCI. Card Interv TODAY 2019;13(1):44–8.
6. Myat A, Patel N, Tehrani S, et al. Percutaneous circulatory assist devices for high-risk coronary intervention. JACC Cardiovasc Interv 2015;8(2):229–44.
7. Parissis H, Graham V, Lampridis S, et al. IABP: History-evolution-pathophysiology-indications: What we need to know. J Cardiothorac Surg 2016;11(1):122.
8. Jacobey JA. Results of counterpulsation in patients with coronary artery disease. Am J Cardiol 1971;27(2):137–45.
9. De Waha S, Desch S, Eitel I, et al. Intra-aortic balloon counterpulsation - Basic principles and clinical evidence. Vascul Pharmacol 2014;60(2):52–6.
10. Santa-Cruz RA, Cohen MG, Ohman EM. Aortic counterpulsation: A review of the hemodynamic effects and indications for use. Catheter Cardiovasc Interv 2006;67(1):68–77.
11. Zeymer U, Bauer T, Hamm C, et al. Use and impact of intra-aortic balloon pump on mortality in patients with acute myocardial infarction complicated by cardiogenic shock: Results of the Euro Heart Survey on PCI. EuroIntervention 2011;7(4):437–41.
12. Khalid L, Dhakam SH. A Review of Cardiogenic Shock in Acute Myocardial Infarction. Vol 4. 2008. Available at: https://www.ncbi.nlm.nih.gov/pmc/articles/PMC2774583/pdf/CCR-4-34.pdf. Accessed June 30, 2019.
13. Briguori C, Sarais C, Pagnotta P, et al. Elective versus provisional intra-aortic balloon pumping in high-risk percutaneous transluminal coronary angioplasty. Am Heart J 2003;145(4):700–7.
14. Stone GW, Ohman EM, Miller MF, et al. Acute myocardial ischemia/infarction contemporary utilization and outcomes of intra-aortic balloon counterpulsation in acute myocardial infarction the benchmark registry. J Am Coll Cardiol 2003. https://doi.org/10.1016/S0735-1097(03)00400-5.
15. Neumann FJ, Sousa-Uva M, Ahlsson A, et al. 2018 ESC/EACTS Guidelines on myocardial revascularization. Eur Heart J 2019;40(2):87–165.
16. O'Gara PT, Kushner FG, Ascheim DD, et al. 2013 ACCF/AHA guideline for the management of st-elevation myocardial infarction: A report of the American college of cardiology foundation/american heart association task force on practice guidelines. J Am Coll Cardiol 2013;61(4):78–140.
17. Amin AP, Spertus JA, Curtis JP, et al. The evolving landscape of impella use in the United States among patients undergoing percutaneous coronary intervention with mechanical circulatory support. Circulation 2020;273–84.
18. Remmelink M, Sjauw KD, Henriques JPS, et al. Effects of left ventricular unloading by Impella recover LP2.5 on coronary hemodynamics. Catheter Cardiovasc Interv 2007;70(4):532–7.
19. Remmelink M, Sjauw KD, Henriques JPS, et al. Effects of mechanical left ventricular unloading by impella on left ventricular dynamics in high-risk and primary percutaneous coronary intervention patients. Catheter Cardiovasc Interv 2010;75(2):187–94.

20. Greenbaum AB, Babaliaros VC, Chen MY, et al. Transcaval access and closure for transcatheter aortic valve replacement: a prospective investigation. J Am Coll Cardiol 2017;69(5):511–21.

21. O'Neill WW, Kleiman NS, Moses J, et al. A prospective, randomized clinical trial of hemodynamic support with impella 2.5 versus intra-aortic balloon pump in patients undergoing high-risk percutaneous coronary intervention: The PROTECT II study. Circulation 2012. Doi: 10.1161/CIRCULATIO-NAHA.112.098194.

22. Kovacic JC, Nguyen HT, Karajgikar R, et al. The impella recover 2.5 and TandemHeart ventricular assist devices are safe and associated with equivalent clinical outcomes in patients undergoing high-risk percutaneous coronary intervention. Catheter Cardiovasc Interv 2013;82(1):E28–37.

23. Burkhoff D, Cohen H, Brunckhorst C, et al. A randomized multicenter clinical study to evaluate the safety and efficacy of the TandemHeart percutaneous ventricular assist device versus conventional therapy with intraaortic balloon pumping for treatment of cardiogenic shock. Am Heart J 2006;152(3):469.e1-e8.

24. Kar B, Gregoric ID, Basra SS, et al. The Percutaneous Ventricular Assist Device in Severe Refractory Cardiogenic Shock. J Am Coll Cardiol 2011. https://doi.org/10.1016/j.jacc.2010.08.613.

25. Reversal of Cardiogenic Shock by Percutaneous Left Atrial-to-Femoral Arterial Bypass Assistance | Ovid. Available at: https://oce.ovid.com/article/00003017-200112110-00035. Accessed April 11, 2020.

26. Teirstein PS, Vogel RA, Vandormael MG, et al. Prophylactic Versus Standby Cardiopulmonary Support for High Risk Percutaneous Transluminal Coronary Angioplasty. J Am Coll Cardiol 1993; 21(3):590–6.

27. Sheu J-J, Tsai T-H, Lee F-Y, et al. Early extracorporeal membrane oxygenator-assisted primary percutaneous coronary intervention improved 30-day clinical outcomes in patients with ST-segment elevation myocardial infarction complicated with profound cardiogenic shock. Crit Care Med 2010; 38(9):1810–7.

28. Basir MB, Schreiber T, Dixon S, et al. Feasibility of early mechanical circulatory support in acute myocardial infarction complicated by cardiogenic shock: The Detroit cardiogenic shock initiative. Catheter Cardiovasc Interv 2018;91(3):454–61.

29. Ostadal P, Rokyta R, Kruger A, et al. Extra corporeal membrane oxygenation in the therapy of cardiogenic shock (ECMO-CS): rationale and design of the multicenter randomized trial. Eur J Heart Fail 2017;19:124–7.

30. Korabathina R, Heffernan KS, Paruchuri V, et al. The pulmonary artery pulsatility index identifies severe right ventricular dysfunction in acute inferior myocardial infarction. Catheter Cardiovasc Interv 2012;80(4):593–600.

31. Morine KJ, Kiernan MS, Pham DT, et al. Pulmonary artery pulsatility index is associated with right ventricular failure after left ventricular assist device surgery. J Card Fail 2016;22(2):110–6.

32. Zehender M, Kasper W, Kauder E, et al. Right ventricular infarction as an independent predictor of prognosis after acute inferior myocardial infarction. N Engl J Med 1993;328(14):981–8.

33. Haddad F, Doyle R, Murphy DJ, et al. Right ventricular function in cardiovascular disease, part II: Pathophysiology, clinical importance, and management of right ventricular failure. Circulation 2008;117(13): 1717–31.

34. ABIOMED | Impella RP®. Available at: http://www. abiomed.com/impella/impella-rp. Accessed April 21, 2020.

35. Anderson M, Morris L, Tang D, et al. Impella RP Post Approval Study: First Multi-Center, Prospective Post Market Approval Results for the Impella RP in Patients with Right Ventricular Failure. J Heart Lung Transplant 2017;36(4):S64–5.

36. Cheung AW, White CW, Davis MK, et al. Short-term mechanical circulatory support for recovery from acute right ventricular failure: Clinical outcomes. J Heart Lung Transplant 2014;33(8):794–9.

37. Anderson MB, Goldstein J, Milano C, et al. Benefits of a novel percutaneous ventricular assist device for right heart failure: The prospective RECOVER RIGHT study of the Impella RP device. J Heart Lung Transplant 2015;34(12):1549–60.

38. Post-Approval Studies (PAS). Available at: https:// www.accessdata.fda.gov/scripts/cdrh/cfdocs/ cfpma/pma_pas.cfm?t_id=615919&c_id=4556. Accessed August 17, 2020.

39. Nicolais CD, Suryapalam M, O'Murchu B, et al. Use of protek duo tandem heart for percutaneous right ventricular support in various clinical settings: a case series. J Am Coll Cardiol 2018; 71(11):A1314.

40. Ravichandran AK, Baran DA, Stelling K, et al. Outcomes with the tandem protek duo dual-lumen percutaneous right ventricular assist device. ASAIO J 2018;64(4):570–2.

41. Tehrani BN, Truesdell AG, Sherwood MW, et al. Standardized Team-Based Care for Cardiogenic Shock. J Am Coll Cardiol 2019;73(13). https://doi. org/10.1016/j.jacc.2018.12.084.

42. Mazimba S, Kennedy JLW, Zhuo D, et al. Decreased pulmonary arterial proportional pulse pressure after pulmonary artery catheter optimization for advanced heart failure is associated with adverse clinical outcomes. J Card Fail 2016; 22(12). https://doi.org/10.1016/j.cardfail.2016.03. 019.

43. Marcolino MS, Simsek C, De Boer SPM, et al. Short- and long-term outcomes in octogenarians undergoing percutaneous coronary intervention with stenting. EuroIntervention 2012;8(8):920–8.

44. Batchelor WB, Anstrom KJ, Muhlbaier LH, et al. Contemporary Outcome Trends in the Elderly Undergoing Percutaneous Coronary Interventions: Results in 7,472 Octogenarians. J Am Coll Cardiol 2000;36(3):723–30.

45. Abaunza M, Kabbani LS, Nypaver T, et al. From the Midwestern Vascular Surgical Society Incidence and prognosis of vascular complications after percutaneous placement of left ventricular assist device. J Vasc Surg 2015;62:417–23.

46. Ouweneel DM, Eriksen E, Sjauw KD, et al. Percutaneous Mechanical Circulatory Support Versus Intra-Aortic Balloon Pump in Cardiogenic Shock After Acute Myocardial Infarction. J Am Coll Cardiol 2017;69(3):278–87.

47. Goldberg RJ, Spencer FA, Gore JM, et al. Thirty-year trends (1975 to 2005) in the magnitude of, management of, and hospital death rates associated with cardiogenic shock in patients with acute myocardial infarction a population-based perspective. Circulation 2009;119(9):1211–9.

48. Percutaneous left ventricular assist devices vs intra-aortic balloon pump counterpulsation for treatment of cardiogenic shock: a meta-analysis of controlled trials - Database of Abstracts of Reviews of Effects (DARE): Quality-assessed Reviews - NCBI Bookshelf. Available at: https://www.ncbi.nlm.nih.gov/books/NBK77141/. Accessed April 25, 2020.

When Things Get Stuck
Gear Entrapment and Other Complications of Chronic Total Occlusion Percutaneous Coronary Intervention

Stewart Benton Jr, MD[a], William J. Nicholson, MD[b],*

KEYWORDS

- Gear entrapment • Fracture • Embolization • Chronic total occlusion • Complications

KEY POINTS

- Meticulous procedural planning is essential to mitigate the risks of complications an equipment failure. Despite preparation, device failure, fracture and entrapment will occur.
- Appropriate vessel preparation and understanding the limitations of equipment is essential for avoiding gear failure and entrapment.
- The complex coronary artery operator must have a structured algorithm for assessing the mechanism of gear failure and entrapment with a stepwise approach to how to solve the problem.

The greater the difficulty, the more glory in surmounting it. Skillful pilots gain their reputation from storms and tempests.
—Epictetus

INTRODUCTION

Revascularization of chronic total occlusions (CTO) is a complex undertaking increased risk of complications compared with routine percutaneous coronary intervention (PCI). Risk can be mitigated by careful preparation and meticulous procedural technique; however, all complications cannot be avoided.[1] Therefore, operators must be aware of their possibility and management strategies. This article focuses on complications encountered during CTO PCI, which are not addressed elsewhere in this issue. The information has been organized to present a structured framework through which procedural complications may be identified and managed. However, the recommendations offered in this article represent cumulative operator experience and not randomized data that are lacking in this subject. Therefore, clinical judgment and operator discretion are encouraged.

Intraprocedural complications of CTO PCI are listed in Fig. 1.[1,2] Coronary complications include acute vessel closure, perforation, and equipment failure (loss/entrapment). This article focuses on the diagnosis and management of equipment failure, myocardial ischemia, and noncardiac complications. The management of coronary perforation is discussed elsewhere. This article focuses on the technical aspects of complication avoidance, recognition, and management.

The prevention of complications is far preferable to complication management. Careful procedural planning and commitment to technical fundamentals are required before undertaking any complex intervention. Listed as follows are

[a] Interventional Cardiology, Wellspan York Hospital, 25 Monument Road, Suite 200, York, PA 17403, USA;
[b] Interventional Cardiology, Complex Coronary and Cardiac Intervention, Emory University, Suite F606, 1364 Clifton Road, Atlanta, GA 30322, USA
* Corresponding author.
E-mail address: wjnicho@emory.edu

Intervent Cardiol Clin 10 (2021) 131–145
https://doi.org/10.1016/j.iccl.2020.09.007

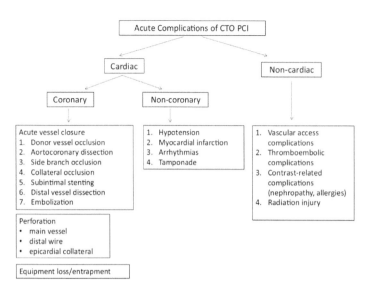

Fig. 1. Intraprocedural complications of CTO PCI.

5 important steps in mitigating the risk of complications.

1. Know the anatomy: Carefully review the angiogram before the procedure and adopt a procedural approach as directed by the hybrid algorithm.[3,4] Note the presence of heavy calcification, tortuosity, and existing stents along the pathway of equipment delivery. Be prepared to move laterally within the hybrid algorithm as procedural impasses arise.
2. Know your equipment: Have a thorough understanding of equipment design and understand how the specific properties of each tool dictate its use and limitations.
3. Anticipate difficulty and set up for success: Routine use of 45-cm-long sheaths from the femoral approach is recommended. Coaxial engagement of supportive, 7-Fr or 8-Fr guide catheters at the beginning of the case will increase procedural efficacy and efficiency.
4. Prepare the vessel: Adequate vessel preparation is key to optimizing stent results and to mitigating the risk of equipment failure. Proactive vessel preparation is safer and more efficient than prolonged trial and error approaches that may lead to complications.
5. Focus on technical fundamentals: Meticulous procedural technique is required to avoid complications. Several fundamental principles for effective procedural technique are listed in Box 1.

Despite these efforts, procedural complications may still occur. The following segments will address specific complications encountered during CTO PCI and their management.

EQUIPMENT FAILURE

Despite substantial improvements in CTO equipment design and engineering, equipment failure may still occur. The 3 main mechanisms of equipment failure are entrapment, fracture, and loss or embolization. The patient and procedural characteristics that increase the risk of equipment failure are listed in Fig. 2.[2,5,6]

General Management of Equipment Failure
The fundamental steps of equipment failure management are described in Fig. 3. This algorithm is applicable to the management of entrapment or fracture of all coronary equipment. In the event of equipment failure, it is important to first maintain the fundamentals of coronary intervention. One procedural complication may be managed; however, compounding complications inflicted during failed management attempts is often disastrous. A simple, efficient approach to complication management is often best.

Avoid losing wire position and maintain therapeutic activated clotting times throughout the procedure. It is of critical importance that the operator understands the mechanism of equipment failure. This requires complete visualization of the coronary tree, a full inspection of the guide catheter, and a working knowledge of

Coronary Guidewire:

Avoid excessive torque when a wire tip is
engaged in the CTO segment or the
subintimal space.

Never spin a knuckled wire. Once a wire is
knuckled, it should only be advanced or
retracted.

Jail jacketed wires when necessary; do not jail
nonjacketed wires.

Coronary Stents:

Do not attempt to deliver a stent through
side struts of an existing stent that have not
been predilated.

Always stent distally to proximally.

Proactive use of guide extensions will
mitigate the risk of stent deformation and
stent loss.

Microcatheter:

Never torque or advance a microcatheter
without a guidewire in place distally.

If the microcatheter is not advancing, do not
continue to apply torque as this may lead to
tip fracture.

Limit the rotations of a microcatheter in a
single direction to 10 or fewer, then reverse
torque.

When advancing microcatheters, ensure the
guide is engaged, the system is straight, and
there is adequate distal wire purchase for
support.

Avoiding Entrapment:

Avoid mating of antegrade and retrograde
gear on the same externalized wire.

Never jail an externalized guidewire.

Never snare the stiff portion of a wire that is
intended to be externalized as this will kink
the wire after it is pulled into the retrograde
guide potentially resulting in total equipment
entrapment.

the equipment used. Finally, the anatomic location of equipment failure should be considered, as this is likely to direct management.

The 2 principal mechanisms of equipment failure are entrapment and fracture. In the case of entrapment, a piece of coronary equipment becomes lodged in the coronary artery and resists traditional efforts at removal. Great caution is required when pulling entrapped equipment,

as the force applied will be transmitted to the guide catheter. This can result in unintentional deep engagement of the guide and vessel dissection. Injury to the proximal vessel may also occur if an uncovered wire or balloon shaft is pulled forcefully. Therefore, it is preferable to advance a microcatheter or guide extension over entrapped equipment when possible.[7]

Entrapment typically occurs due to interaction between a heavily diseased segment of the vessel and the wire, microcatheter, or balloon. However, all coronary equipment including atherectomy devices and imaging catheters may become entrapped. To free the equipment, the 3-dimensional relationship between the artery and device must be altered. There are several strategies available to the operator that are outlined in Fig. 3. In some cases, straightening of the coronary artery from the passage of a supportive buddy wire is all that is required to free entrapped equipment. Once parallel wiring is achieved, balloon techniques may be performed. Balloon inflation adjacent to the entrapped equipment is often effective at facilitating removal. In some cases, it may be preferable to deliver a small balloon distally and drag the inflated balloon back to the site of entrapment. The interaction between the balloon and the distal site of entrapment may free the device. This balloon-drag technique is also effective in cases of equipment fracture or embolization. If fracture has not occurred, or if a fractured segment remains partially in the coronary guide catheter, a balloon may be inflated in the guide to trap or pin the equipment to the guide. Attempts can then be made to remove the guide, balloon, and entrapped equipment as a unit.

If these steps are unsuccessful, or if a parallel wire cannot be successfully delivered distal to the site of entrapment, then retrieval efforts can continue by using snares to grasp the equipment in the distal guide. Force transmission is greater when pulling from a snare compared with pulling from the distal end of the entrapped equipment. If a snare is not available, then the braided wires technique may be used in which 2 wires are delivered parallel to the entrapped equipment and spun rapidly. The distal ends of the wires should be fed through a single torquer to facilitate this maneuver. The wires will become entangled with the entrapped equipment providing extra support and force during removal attempts.[8] Finally, if these techniques have failed, a wire can be used to access the subintimal space proximal to the site of entrapment. Ballooning of the subintimal space may alter the vessel architecture enough to free the

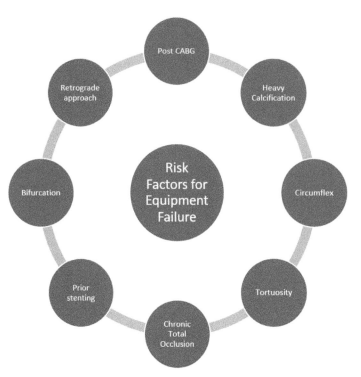

Fig. 2. Clinical and morphologic characteristics that predispose equipment to failure.

entrapped equipment. However, before using subintimal techniques, consideration must be given to the likelihood of gaining successful reentry to the true lumen and to the potential loss of side branches.

In the case of equipment fracture, many of the same techniques are applicable. However, the initial step is to identify the location of the retained fragment relative to the coronary artery and guide catheter. If a portion of the fragment is retained in the guide, balloon trapping may be used to recover the fractured segment. If the fragment is not retained in the guide, then parallel wiring should be performed, and a guide

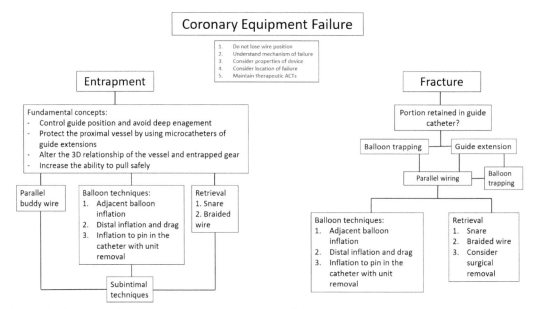

Fig. 3. Fundamentals of equipment management to prevent failure.

extension catheter delivered over top of the fragment. Balloon trapping may then be attempted in the guide extension. Once a parallel wire is delivered distal to the fragment, the "balloon-drag" technique may be used. Retrieval attempts can include the use of snares or the braided wire technique if the fragment is not located in the guide, if the fragment cannot be captured in a guide extension, and if parallel wiring is unsuccessful. In extreme cases of entrapment or fracture, surgical removal may be considered as a final option.[6,9]

Specific Scenarios
Wire failure
The incidence of wire failure in CTO PCI is greater than that of routine PCI due to the complexity of disease encountered in this patient population and the extreme demands often placed on wires for successful CTO crossing. Although a comprehensive review of coronary guidewire engineering is beyond the scope of this article, there are several key concepts of wire design that merit review.

Wire design. Coronary guidewires consist of 4 components: a core element, body, tip, and coating. The central core element of the wire is steel, nitinol, or a combination of both. The core element may extend the length of the wire or stop several millimeters short of the distal tip in which case a shaping ribbon is used. The core element tapers as it nears the distal wire tip. The body of the wire consists of coils or polymers that surround the core element. Many wires feature a hybrid design with a polymer covering most of the wire and coils covering the distal tip. The body of the wire is then sprayed with a hydrophilic or hydrophobic coating.[10]

The tip of the wire is typically composed of coils that may be exposed or covered with a polytetrafluoroethylene (PTFE) sleeve or jacket. Exposed, nonjacketed coils at the wire tip enhance shape retention, one-to-one torque transmission, and tactile feedback. However, this is at the expense of lubricity. Conversely, jacketed wires are highly lubricious but lack tip durability, tactile feedback, and torque transmission. Therefore, composite core (or dual core) technology was introduced to overcome such limitations. Composite core wires feature a twist wire and traditional core element that, together, form the functional core of the wire.[11] The 2 elements run the length of the wire. The core and twist wire are then jointly wrapped by a third rope wire that terminates before the distal tip.

This design greatly enhances torque transmission and wire durability despite the presence or absence of a jacketed tip.

Mechanisms of wire failure. These design elements are important when considering mechanisms of wire failure, which include entrapment, fracture, and unraveling of wire components. Coronary guidewire entrapment may occur due to severe vessel calcification or tortuosity and interactions between the guidewire and other pieces of coronary equipment such a microcatheter or stent struts. Entrapment may also result from errors in technique. Guidewire fracture typically results from overrotation of the wire and increased torsional stress. The distal 3 cm of most coronary wires represent a point of mechanical weakness that is often implicated as the site of wire fracture.[6,12–14] If excessive force is applied pulling an entrapped wire the coils may unravel from the core. This can result in entanglement of large amounts of material in the coronary artery and aorta precluding percutaneous removal. Knowledge of wire design is also important when inspecting an entrapped wire after successful removal. Close evaluation of each wire segment should be performed to ensure no wire components are unknowingly left in the vessel or embolized during wire retrieval.

Common scenarios implicated in wire failure. Independent of wire design, there are certain maneuvers that increase the risk of wire entrapment and fracture that must be carefully navigated or avoided entirely. Wire pinning behind stent struts (jailing) may lead to entrapment or fracture. Only hydrophilic, polymer jacketed wires should be jailed. Minor structural damage to the jacket may occur. However, nonjacketed wires routinely suffer major structural damage and risk coil unraveling after being jailed.[15]

Overrotation of a guidewire when the tip is engaged in a CTO segment will result in disproportionate torsional stress applied to the wire proximal to the tip. This can lead to wire fracture and unraveling of core components. A similar scenario can result if a subintimal wire is aggressively torqued over 180°. During CTO crossing, careful attention must be payed to ensure that torque applied to the wire is being transmitted to the tip.[16]

Subintimal techniques require formation of a knuckle to facilitate blunt dissection and lesion crossing. It is important to never spin a knuckled wire. This can result in wire fracture or knot formation of the distal wire tip. If a knot forms, it may be very difficult to retrieve the wire without fracture of the distal segment and unraveling of the subcomponents of the wire.

Several specialty wires have been designed for collateral crossing during the retrograde approach. These wires typically have low gram weighted tips which are less traumatic and more compliant. These wires should not be spun due to the possibility that the tip can loop onto itself and form a knot. This makes further navigation across the collateral impossible and complicates wire retrieval, often damaging the collateral vessel in the process. Therefore, when using low tip weighted wires, the tip should be kept free during collateral traversal but not rotated over 90 to 180°.[17]

During retrograde CTO PCI, the retrograde wire is directed into the antegrade guide for externalization. However, if the antegrade guide or guide extension cannot be successfully wired, the retrograde wire can be snared through an antegrade guide for the purposes of externalization. Dedicated externalization wires should be preferentially snared. The stiff portion of the wire should not be snared and pulled into the antegrade guide. This will form a kink in the wire and lock the wire and snare together such that the wire cannot be released and separated from the snare while still in the body. If unforeseen resistance is encountered during efforts to complete externalization of the snared wire, total equipment entrapment may result.[7] This situation leaves the operator with the only solution of cutting the distal portion of the retrograde microcatheter and wire. The operator must then pull the system through the retrograde guide, and the heart and finally out of the antegrade guide.

Wire entrapment. It is helpful to divide management strategies by the mechanism of wire failure. In the case of wire entrapment, management strategies are further subdivided by clinical scenarios: jailed wire, tortuosity, heavy calcification/CTO lesion. Regardless of the mode of entrapment, always avoid excessively pulling on the guidewire. This can cause wire fracture, unraveling of the components of the wire, and injury to the vessel upstream of the entrapment site by the wire itself or from interaction with the guide catheter.

If a wire is entrapped in a vessel due to excessive tortuosity, it is useful to administer intracoronary nitroglycerin to alleviate vessel spasm, if present. This alone may be enough to enable successful removal. If the vessel is otherwise free of significant disease, a low-profile microcatheter should be advanced over the wire and used to facilitate wire removal. This will allow for better translation of force to the long axis of the wire when pulling and provide protection for the proximal vessel. If the wire is entrapped in a tortuous epicardial collateral, anticipate that removal attempts may result in injury or perforation.

If the wire is jailed behind or between deployed stents or entrapped in heavy calcification/CTO segment, the first step is to advance a microcatheter over the wire to the site of entrapment. This allows for better translation of force along the long axis of the wire and may be enough to free the entrapped wire segment. If this fails, exchange the microcatheter for a low-profile balloon. Advance the balloon to the site of entrapment, perform a low-pressure balloon inflation, and reattempt wire removal. If the entrapped wire is jailed, the main vessel stent will need to be post dilated after wire removal to ensure there is no stent deformation.

If this technique fails, remove the balloon and place a guide extension catheter for better support. Repeat steps 1 and 2 for continued retrieval efforts. If this is unsuccessful, you may need to apply more direct force to the distal portion of the wire near the site of entrapment. In this case, pass a snare over the wire and through the guide extension catheter. Grasp the wire upstream from the site of the entrapment and repeat efforts at wire removal.

If these measures fail and the wire is entrapped in a heavily calcified lesion or CTO segment, then subintimal techniques may be useful. A second wire may be used to enter the subintimal space proximal to the site of entrapment. A knuckled wire may then be advanced distal to the entrapped wire, and the lesion modified by ballooning in the subintimal space adjacent to the site of entrapment. This approach can be used from the antegrade guide in the event of retrograde wire entrapment. However, if subintimal techniques are used, the operator should be proficient with reentry techniques and the anatomy should be carefully considered for potential loss of side branches.

If these percutaneous options have failed, then surgical removal should be considered.[15] If the patient is not a surgical candidate, and the wire is still entrapped, one last percutaneous option remains. Pass a new wire over a microcatheter parallel to the entrapped wire. Use the microcatheter to exchange for a Rotafloppy wire. Next, use a rotational atherectomy burr to cut the entrapped wire. Negative traction should be applied to the entrapped wire while atherectomy runs are performed. Once the wire is cut, the retained segment should be excluded from circulation by jailing with stents.[18] Intravascular imaging should be performed to ensure all elements of the retained wire have been covered and that no additional material remains.[19]

Wire fracture. There are 3 main options for management of a fractured guidewire: percutaneous removal, surgical removal, and conservative management or leaving the retained segment in place. The first step in management of guidewire fracture is to assess for uncoiling or unraveling of wire components. Fine coils may be difficult to see on angiography, and intracoronary imaging with intravascular ultrasound or optical coherence tomography can be helpful to assess for smaller wire fragments. Next, the exact anatomic location of the retained material should be defined as this will inform management. The removed wire segment should be carefully inspected. It is helpful to open a new wire for comparison to gain a better understanding of the retained material.

If significant uncoiling has occurred, then there are limited options for full percutaneous retrieval. A snare may be used over a guide extension catheter to attempt retrieval of the wire fragments. However, coils and components of dual core wires are thin and very long when unraveled. They may become intertwined or looped forming a "birds-nest" of retained material in the coronary artery or aorta, which can be very thrombogenic and impossible to retrieve percutaneously.[6] Surgical removal may be required in these scenarios. However, if the patient is not a surgical candidate, the retained material may be excluded from the circulation by jailing with stents. In the situation of unraveled coils, placement of a covered stent should be considered as the retained material may protrude through the struts of open cell stents and function as a nidus for thrombus stent thrombosis. If the wire remnants are entirely confined to a side branch, and if the side branch is not of critical importance, then placement of a covered stent across the bifurcation to exclude the retained material may be a suitable option.

If significant uncoiling has not occurred, then the next step is to establish if the retained segment extends back into the aorta or if it is limited to the coronary artery. If the wire fragment extends beyond the ostium of the coronary, and if it remains in the guide catheter, then balloon trapping should be performed within the guide to facilitate removal as a unit. If the retained wire fragment extends beyond the coronary ostia and is no longer in the guide catheter, then attempts to snare the wire should be made. Once snared, the guide catheter, snare, and wire fragment should be removed as a unit.

If the retained wire fragment does not extend beyond the coronary ostia, then retrieval and abandonment are 2 available management strategies. The anatomic location of the retained fragment should be considered. If the retained material is in a critical location (left main or proximal left anterior descending), management should be focused on retrieval. However, if the wire fragment is in a noncritical branch vessel, then the risks of retrieval should be weight against the risk of abandoning the segment. Retrieval techniques include snaring, aggressively seating the guide to extend to the wire fragment and balloon trapping within the catheter, and the braided wire technique. Fig. 4 is an algorithm for management of wire failure during CTO PCI.

Microcatheter failure
Microcatheter design and application. CTO PCI should always be performed using an over-the-wire system to allow for easy reshaping of the wire tip, efficient wire exchanges, to protect the proximal vessel from guidewire injury and enhance the penetrating force of the wire. This may be accomplished using either a microcatheter or over-the-wire balloon. Microcatheters are preferred as the radiopaque tip allows for accurate catheter location, they have improved trackability compared with balloons, they facilitate guidewire access to angulated side branches, and they have less tendency to kink than do over-the-wire balloons. Microcatheters have many additional functions in contemporary CTO PCI including tip injections for plaque modification, selective contrast injection of collateral branches, and local delivery of fat, thrombin, or coils in case of perforation.[11] Much like coronary guidewires, a basic understanding of microcatheter design will help the operator with microcatheter selection and inform the management of equipment failure.

Microcatheters typically have a body made of a stainless-steel braided mesh, coils, or both. They routinely have an inner lining of PTFE to facilitate wire manipulation and an outer hydrophilic polymer coating to enhance delivery. The body of the microcatheter is joined to a distal tip which is typically tapered and flexible to facilitate atraumatic vessel crossing. Currently

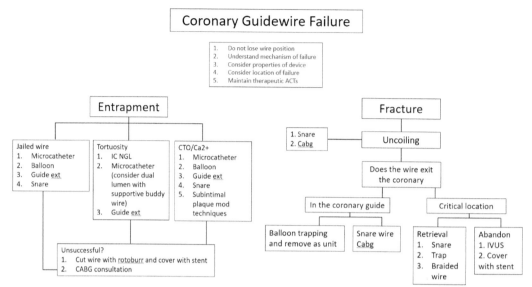

Fig. 4. Management algorithm for wire failure in CTO PCI.

available microcatheters have unique design features intended for specific clinical scenarios such as enhanced antegrade support or improved retrograde collateral crossing (http://asahi-intec-cusa-medical.com/medical-product/corsair-microcatheter/ and https://www.terumois.com/products/catheters/finecross.html).

Microcatheter failure and management: fatigue, tip fracture, and equipment entrapment. A common mechanism of failure is microcatheter fatigue. This results from prolonged use and excessive torqueing of the microcatheter. If fatigue is not detected early, irreversible wire entrapment may occur due to binding of the microcatheter to unraveled components of the wire (Fig. 5). This requires removal of the microcatheter and coronary guidewire as a unit, losing whatever progress had been made. Therefore, it is important to anticipate microcatheter fatigue and to exchange for new equipment proactively. Signs

of microcatheter fatigue include difficulty directing and manipulating the guidewire, difficultly transmitting torque to the microcatheter, and difficulty advancing and withdrawing the microcatheter.[20,21]

Tip fracture is also a well-described mechanism of microcatheter failure. This typically occurs when the tip of a microcatheter is encased within the CTO segment and the body of the microcatheter is continually torqued. Much like with wire fracture, this results in increased torsional stress on the junction of the body of the microcatheter and the distal tip which can cause fracture. Tip fracture occurs more frequently in lower profile, braided mesh microcatheters which are not designed to be aggressively torqued.

If tip fracture occurs, there are several management options. The most important initial step is to maintain wire position. If the fractured tip remains on the wire, a small (1 mm or 1.25 mm) balloon may be advanced into, or

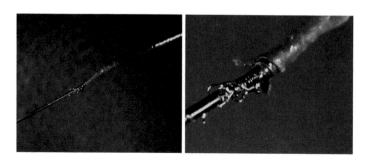

Fig. 5. Binding of the microcatheter and guidewire from excessive torqueing and fatigue of the microcatheter.

distal to, the fractured tip. Low-pressure balloon inflation can be performed to pin or trap the tip for retraction into the guide catheter. Retrieval attempts may be aided by aggressively seating the guide or using a guide extension catheter to minimize the distance required to recapture the fractured tip. Once the fracture tip is in the guide, a second balloon can be used to trap the tip inside the guide catheter to minimize the risk of embolization during removal.

If wire position is lost, the strategies available for tip retrieval are similar to those used in the event of wire fracture. If the microcatheter tip can be captured within the guide catheter or a guide extension, trapping techniques can be used. If these measures are not successful, or if the tip is in the mid or distal segments of the vessel, use of a snare or braided wire technique may be successful. Finally, if the fractured tip is retained in the CTO segment, jailing the fragment with a stent or proceeding with dissection reentry techniques to complete the case and exclude the tip are effective alternatives.

Retrograde techniques routinely require the simultaneous delivery and manipulation of microcatheters and balloons over both antegrade and retrograde limbs of the externalized wires. It is important to never allow the tip of an antegrade microcatheter, balloon, or stent to meet or interact with the tip of the retrograde microcatheter. This may result in mating of the equipment and entrapment. Traditionally, this has been described in the Corsair and Tornus microcatheters. Current generation microcatheters, however, have not been as frequently implicated. In bench testing, mating of the Turnpike family of microcatheters with standard balloons or with microcatheters from the same family did not occur. However, the Corsair Pro and Corsair Pro XS were mated with traditional balloons and with each other resulting in complete entrapment. The best practice is to always avoid meeting of antegrade and retrograde gear (Fig. 6).

Guide catheter extensions

The use of guide catheter extensions has greatly improved the success and efficiency of CTO PCI, and they are essential tools in contemporary practice.[22] Like wires and microcatheters, knowledge of the equipment will mitigate risk and help manage potential complications.

There are multiple guide catheter extensions available in the United States: Guideliner V3 (Vascular Solutions, Minneapolis, MN), Guidezilla II (Boston Scientific, Marlborough, MA), Trapliner (Vascular Solutions), and Telescope (Medtronic, Dublin, Ireland). All guide catheter extensions consist of a push rod and a distal cylinder of variable length (25 cm in the GuideLiner V3 and the Guidezilla II, and 13 cm in the Trapliner and 21 cm in Telescope). They are manufactured in various Fr sizes which, when paired with a guide catheter, result in an inner luminal diameter that is approximately 2 Fr sizes smaller than that of the guide catheter. In addition to the rod and cylinder, the Trapliner also has a balloon proximal to the entry collar that allows trapping of equipment to facilitate exchanges.[11]

There are several potential complications that must be avoided when using guide extensions. A common frustration is the tendency of the guidewire to wrap around the guide extension shaft. This results in failure to deliver coronary balloons or stents and/or loss of wire position when removing equipment. To avoid this scenario, the guide catheter extension push rod should be set away from the path of the coronary wire(s) and to the side of the Y-connector. The distal end of the guide extension is not tapered, and it can easily lift a coronary plaque and cause vessel dissection if advanced into the coronary in an unguided fashion. Delivery over a balloon or microcatheter forms a more stable rail and is preferred to advancement over a coronary wire alone.

If using a guide extension smaller than the guide catheter (6 Fr extension in an 8 Fr guide), wire the vessel first and then advance the guide

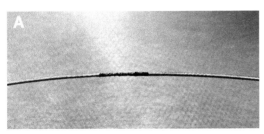 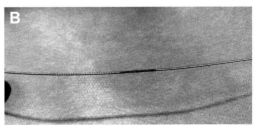

Fig. 6. (A) Mating and entrapment of a microcatheters on a wire and (B) deformation of the tips of microcatheters on a wire. However, mating and entrapment did not occur.

extension over the wire. Avoid attempts to deliver a guidewire in the setting of guide extension/guide catheter mismatch, as the wire may advance between the wall of the guide and the cylinder of the guide extension leading to damage of the wire tip. Deformation of stents or other equipment can occur during advancement through the guide catheter extension collar. To avoid this, it may be necessary to advance the stent or other equipment into the guide extension catheter outside the body and advance both as a single unit over the wire. When introducing new balloons or stents through guide extensions, use fluoroscopic guidance to visualize the stent as it enters the guide catheter extension collar. Deformation of stents or other equipment can occur while withdrawing the equipment back into the distal tip of the extension catheter. Coronary stents should be carefully inspected for damage if removed through a guide extension catheter after failed delivery.

During retrograde interventions, a guide catheter extension can be advanced through the antegrade guide catheter to facilitate reverse controlled antegrade and retrograde tracking and dissection (CART) technique (GuideLiner Reverse CART).[23] Guide catheter extensions may also be used from the retrograde side to increase support for retrograde gear delivery; however, this should be done with care to not injury the donor vessel. Never perform forceful contrast injections with a guide extension catheter extending into the coronary, especially if pressure dampening is present. This can result in significant coronary dissection. In general, placement of guide extensions in donor vessels during CTO PCI should be avoided when possible.

Finally, it is important to note the difference in the length of the cylinders between catheters as the Trapliner is significantly shorter than the GuideLiner and Guidezilla. The proximal collar of the guide catheter extension should never be advanced outside the guide catheter as fracture may occur at the junction of the push rod and cylinder. The proximal end of a fractured push rod is sharp and may cause severe injury to or perforation of the coronary artery or aorta.

Balloon fracture, entrapment, and embolization

Balloon entrapment can occur due to faulty deflation, entanglement and binding of balloon material to stent struts or calcium, or fracture of the delivery shaft. Risk factors for failure are like those of other coronary devices: heavy calcification, tortuosity, bifurcations, and in stent

restenosis. Overuse of a single balloon and increased force on the shaft are risk factors for fracture.[24]

Balloon entrapment may occur if the balloon ruptures and the retained material becomes entangled with vessel calcification or stent struts. Often, the balloon segment may be freed by aggressively seating the guide catheter and by advancing a supportive buddy wire distal to the site of obstruction. This may straighten the vessel and alter the 3-dimensional relationship of the entrapped segment to the vessel and free the balloon. If this is not successful, progressive balloon inflation over the parallel wire may free the entrapped segment. In some cases, subintimal modification of the plaque may be required; however, one should consider the consequences of failed reentry before adopting this strategy.

In the event of balloon fracture, the first fundamental question of the retained gear algorithm is applied: Is a portion retained in the guide catheter or guide extension? If so, then trapping techniques may be used to retrieve the balloon. If this is unsuccessful, a parallel wire should be delivered distal to the retained segment. Previously described balloon strategies for removal such as adjacent ballooning or distal inflation and dragging of the retained segment to the guide may be attempted. If these strategies fail, the balloon fragment can be snared or captured with the braided wire technique for additional retrieval attempts. If the balloon catheter has been successful retrieved with only balloon material remaining in a noncritical anatomic position, then the remaining material may be jailed by stenting. As always, intravascular imaging should be used to ensure all abandoned material is effectively covered.

If, however, the retained segment is not partially in the guide, the location of the retained segment must be carefully considered. Fracture of a balloon shaft results in a sharp, ridged retained fragment that can cause serious injury to the coronary artery and aorta. Therefore, the initial retrieval strategy is to pass a parallel wire distal to the retained fragment and capture the fractured shaft within a guide extension. If the retained segment is located distally in a coronary artery or vein graft, the mother, daughter, granddaughter technique may be required.[25–27] Once the balloon fragment is successfully captured by the guide extension, snaring, balloon trapping, or braided wire techniques can be used for retrieval. If these techniques fail, operative removal may be considered.[28]

Last, balloon rupture is not an uncommon occurrence during CTO interventions. This is an intentional technique used in some circumstances to modify recalcitrant plaques. If a balloon is likely to rupture, it should be meticulously prepped on the table to ensure a continuous fluid column that is free of air. This simple step reduces the risk of vessel perforation and air embolism in the event of rupture.

Stent loss

Stent loss during percutaneous coronary intervention is infrequent with an incidence of approximately 0.3% during routine PCI. The incidence is CTO PCI is not well reported. However, the same risk factors for general equipment failure are also risk factors for stent loss.[29] If an undeployed stent is stripped off the balloon catheter, it is critical for the location of the stent to be assessed quickly. Stripped stents can easily embolize into the distal coronary artery or into the systemic circulation causing stroke or lodging in the peripheral vasculature. There are 3 main strategies in the management of stent loss: retrieval, deployment, and crushing[29–32] (Fig. 7).

Maintaining guidewire position within the lost stent is critical for facilitating retrieval or deployment. Therefore, all efforts should be made to maintain initial wire position. A very effective retrieval strategy is the small balloon technique, in which a low-profile balloon is advanced through and distal to the stent. The balloon is then inflated and withdrawn along with the undeployed stent into the guide catheter and the system removed as a unit. Lost stents can also be retrieved using snares or the braided wire technique. Finally, a parallel wire may be placed and a guide extension used to capture to the stent. Trapping techniques can then be used for retrieval.

If wire position is retained, stent deployment may also be a suitable management strategy. In this technique, the stent is progressively dilated with increasingly large balloons until it is fully deployed. If the stent is significantly smaller than the vessel segment in which it is located, a balloon inflation may be performed to low pressure within the stent and the unit advanced distally to a segment more appropriately sized.

If initial wire position is lost such that the stent is freely embolized in the coronary artery, then retrieval strategies are limited to snaring, the braided wire technique, and capturing the lost stent within a guide extension for the purposes of trapping. If these techniques fail, and if the lost stent is not located in a critical anatomic location, jailing of the stent against the vessel wall by deployment of a new stent is a remaining option.

Rotablator burr entrapment

Severe calcification can be difficult or impossible to adequately dilate with balloon inflations alone and poor preparation results in suboptimal stent expansion, predisposing to restenosis and stent thrombosis. Rotational atherectomy was introduced in 1988 by David Auth and colleagues[33] and is conventionally available as the Rotablator Rotational Atherectomy system (Boston Scientific, https://www.bostonscientific.com/content/gwc/en-US/products/atherectomy-systems/rotational-atherectomy-systems/rotablator.html), which features an advancer to control movement of the burr. The advancer can be purchased

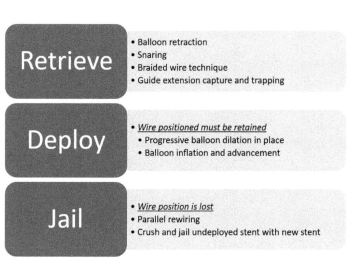

Fig. 7. Three main strategies in the management of stent loss: retrieval, deployment, and crushing.

individually (ROTALink Advancer) or pre-connected to the burr catheter (ROTALink Plus Catheter). Although use of the system is indispensable to adequate vessel preparation, burr entrapment in the target coronary artery is a rare (0.4%) but potentially disastrous complication.[34] The focus of this section is to understand the mechanisms that lead to entrapment to mitigate the risk of its occurrence, and to illustrate potential countermeasures to use if the situation of entrapment occurs.

The mechanisms for burr entrapment can be divided into 3 scenarios. First, tracking the burr from outside the body over the ROTAWire to zone of the vessel requiring atherectomy creates undue forward spring-like force on the system. Upon releasing this forward force and initiating rotablation, the burr is predisposed to rapidly jet forward without adequate initial debulking. As a result, the burr can pass through the lesion and become stuck distal to the calcified segment. Because the diamond impregnated section of the burr is only located on the front half of the burr, atherectomy does not occur when the burr is withdrawn, and the blunt shape of the proximal end of the burr (particularly in the 1.25-mm device) can cause it to become stuck and be unable to be withdrawn. To prevent this, the advancer knob should be tightened down in the retraction position approximately 1 to 2 finger breaths from maximum retraction when delivering the burr through the guide to the proximal vessel. Before initiating rotablation, the advancer knob should be loosened to release the built up spring tension to neutralize the system. In addition, consideration to begin with a 1.5-mm burr is encouraged, as the shape of the 1.25-mm burr makes it more apt to become stuck with the initial atherectomy passes.

The second and third scenarios resulting in burr entrapment occur within the calcified lesion segment of the target vessel. Rapid deceleration of the burr can occur when forceful forward pressure is exerted, resulting in the burr aggressively interacting with calcium. First, this can cause the speed of the burr's rotation to decline to the point that the burr itself becomes lodged in the calcification causing the system to come to a rapid stall. Second, if repetitive aggressive forward force is applied, the drive shaft cable of the system can fail and snap resulting in a loss of any transmission of rotation to the burr. Both scenarios can lead to extreme lodging in the lesion, frequently obliterating the residual lumen of the vessel, leading to coronary occlusion and resultant acute ischemia. The burr should never be allowed to stop spinning within a lesion. During ablation, the operator should be attentive to potential warning signs, which may be visual (lack of smooth advancement under fluoroscopy), auditory (pitch changes with variation in resistance encountered by burr), or tactile (resistance in advancer knob or excessive driveshaft vibration).[35,36]

Regardless of the mechanism of burr entrapment, a series of potential retrieval strategies have been used and reported on in the literature. Placement of a second guidewire past the stuck burr allows the operator to pass progressively larger balloons to allow for inflation next to the burr in an effort to free it from its position. This has been done in both the true lumen of the vessel and also when the second guidewire is placed in the subintimal space to allow subintimal plaque modification adjacent to the stuck burr (Fig. 8). If this is unsuccessful, or if a second guidewire cannot be successfully navigated distal to the entrapped gear, increasing mechanisms of exerting leverage for pulling the burr back are attempted. The distal 2.2 cm of the ROTAWire have an intentional step-up increasing the wire's diameter to 0.014 inch to prevent the accidental passing of the burr off of the distal end of the wire. The junction between the tapered portion of the ROTAWire and this step up is very resilient and can be leveraged to allow the operator to apply extreme forces to pull the lodged burr backward toward the guide catheter. Such a strong pulling force will telescope the guide catheter into the coronary, predisposing the artery to guide induced dissection of the proximal vessel (Fig. 9). The

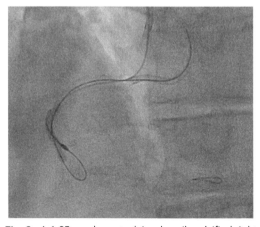

Fig. 8. A 1.25-mm burr stuck in a heavily calcified right coronary artery. A second wire has been advanced into the subintimal space next to the stuck burr to allow adjacent ballooning to dislodge the burr.

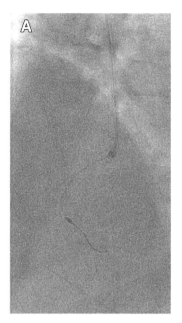
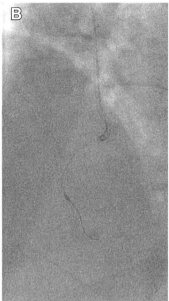

Fig. 9. Extreme forceful negative withdrawal of the stuck burr by leveraging the strong step-up resilience of the distal 2.2 cm of the guidewire. Note the buckling and distress of the guide due to the pulling force.

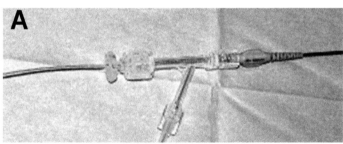
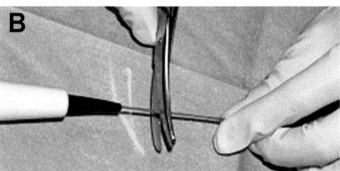
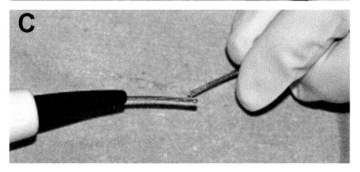

Fig. 10. Cutting the drive shaft cable and wire near the advancer will allow the operator to place a smaller guide, guide catheter extension or goose neck snare over the system to allow telescoping to the lodged burr.

desire to disengage the guide catheter into the aorta must be tempered with the concern of creating a slicing effect of the wire against the coronary-aorta junction. Multiple reports on using a mother-daughter guide catheter configuration, or a guide-catheter extension have been described to assist with this pulling force technique.[37,38] To achieve this, the drive shaft must be cut distal to the advancer (**Fig. 10**), and then the smaller-caliber guide catheter or guide catheter extension can be placed over the drive shaft and advanced down the coronary artery as close to the stuck burr as possible.[39] Using a hemostat to grasp the ROTAWire outside of the body when applying heavy negative withdrawing force avoids having the operator's hand exposed for potential injury from the bare wire.

Additional modifications of these retrieval techniques have been described. Passing of a 4-mm gooseneck micro-snare has been over the ROTAWire and around the burr in a lasso configuration has allowed greater coaxial pulling force, especially when combined with the previously described guide catheter extension technique.[40,41] Finally, there is a case report of placing a second ROTAWire distal to the entrapped burr and utilization of a parallel Rotablator burr to core out the lodged burr.

As with all complications, prevention is always the preferable solution. In the occasion that the previously described techniques for burr dislodgement fail, surgical removal of the entrapped gear is the remaining option when other strategies fail.

SUMMARY

The revascularization of CTOs is a complex undertaking. Careful procedural planning and sound technical fundamentals can mitigate the risk of complications. However, the techniques described in this article should provide effective guidance on the management of equipment failure and entrapment should it occur.

DISCLOSURE

The authors have nothing to disclose.

REFERENCES

1. Brilakis ES, Karmpaliotis D, Patel V, et al. Complications of chronic total occlusion angioplasty. Interv Cardiol Clin 2012;1(3):373–89.
2. Brilakis E. Chapter 12 - Complications. In: Brilakis E, editor. Manual of chronic total occlusion interventions. 2nd Edition. Academic Press; 2018. p. 367–439.
3. Brilakis E. Chapter 7 - Putting it all together: the hybrid approach. In: Brilakis E, editor. Manual of chronic total occlusion interventions. 2nd Edition. Academic Press; 2018. p. 253–65.
4. Brilakis ES, Grantham JA, Rinfret S, et al. A percutaneous treatment algorithm for crossing coronary chronic total occlusions. JACC Cardiovasc Interv 2012;5(4):367–79.
5. Dash D. Complications encountered in coronary chronic total occlusion intervention: Prevention and bailout. Indian Heart J 2016;68(5):737–46.
6. Iturbe JM, Abdel-Karim AR, Papayannis A, et al. Frequency, treatment, and consequences of device loss and entrapment in contemporary percutaneous coronary interventions. J Invasive Cardiol 2012;24(5):215–21.
7. Wu EB, Tsuchikane E. The inherent catastrophic traps in retrograde CTO PCI. Catheter Cardiovasc Interv 2018;91(6):1101–9.
8. Devidutta S, Lim ST. Twisting wire technique: an effective method to retrieve fractured guide wire fragments from coronary arteries. Cardiovasc Revasc Med 2016;17(4):282–6.
9. Azzalini L, Tzanis G, Mashayekhi K, et al. Solving challenging situations and complications in everyday percutaneous coronary intervention using chronic total occlusion techniques. J Invasive Cardiol 2020;32(3):E63–72.
10. Toth GG, Yamane M, Heyndrickx GR. How to select a guidewire: technical features and key characteristics. Heart 2015;101(8):645–52.
11. Brilakis E. Chapter 2 - Equipment. In: Brilakis E, editor. Manual of chronic total occlusion interventions. 2nd Edition. Academic Press; 2018. p. 21–99.
12. Baumann S, Rupp D, Becher T, et al. Retrieval of a fractured angioplasty guidewire after percutaneous retrograde revascularization of coronary chronic total occlusion. Coron Artery Dis 2018;29(1):81–2.
13. Danek BA, Karatasakis A, Brilakis ES. Consequences and treatment of guidewire entrapment and fracture during percutaneous coronary intervention. Cardiovasc Revasc Med 2016;17(2):129–33.
14. Yu CW, Lee HJ, Suh J, et al. Coronary computed tomography angiography predicts guidewire crossing and success of percutaneous intervention for chronic total occlusion: Korean Multicenter CTO CT Registry Score as a tool for assessing difficulty in chronic total occlusion percutaneous coronary intervention. Circ Cardiovasc Imaging 2017; 10(4):e005800.
15. Pan M, Ojeda S, Villanueva E, et al. Structural ial. JACC Cardiovasc Interv 2016;9(18):1917–24.
16. Sianos G, Papafaklis MI. Septal wire entrapment during recanalisation of a chronic total occlusion

with the retrograde approach. Hellenic J Cardiol 2011;52(1):79–83.

17. Park SH, Rha SW, Her K. Retrograde guidewire fracture complicated with pericardial tamponade in chronic total occlusive coronary lesion. Int J Cardiovasc Imaging 2015;31(7):1293–4.

18. Cho JY, Hong SJ. Successful retrieval of entrapped Gaia guidewire in calcified chronic total occlusion using rotational atherectomy device. Int Heart J 2018;59(3):614–7.

19. Corballis N, Sulfi S, Ryding A. optical coherence tomographic study of a chronically retained coronary guidewire. Case Rep Cardiol 2018;2018: 9210764.

20. Karatasakis A, Tarar MN, Karmpaliotis D, et al. Guidewire and microcatheter utilization patterns during antegrade wire escalation in chronic total occlusion percutaneous coronary intervention: Insights from a contemporary multicenter registry. Catheter Cardiovasc Interv 2017;89(4):E90–8.

21. Zhong X, Ge L, Ma J, et al. Microcatheter collateral channel tracking failure in retrograde percutaneous coronary intervention for chronic total occlusion: incidence, predictors, and management. Eurointervention 2019;15(3):e253–60.

22. Tsukui T, Sakakura K, Taniguchi Y, et al. Comparison of the device performance between the conventional guide extension catheter and the soft guide extension catheter. Cardiovasc Revasc Med 2019;20(2):113–9.

23. Xenogiannis I, Karmpaliotis D, Alaswad K, et al. Comparison between traditional and guide-catheter extension reverse controlled antegrade dissection and retrograde tracking: insights from the PROGRESS-CTO Registry. J Invasive Cardiol 2019;31(1):27–34.

24. Nomura T, Higuchi Y, Kato T, et al. A rare instructive complication of balloon catheter fracture during percutaneous coronary intervention. Cardiovasc Interv Ther 2016;31(1):70–4.

25. Kumar P, Aggarwal P, Sinha SK, et al. The safety and efficacy of Guidezilla Catheter (Mother-in-Child Catheter) in complex coronary interventions: an observational study. Cardiol Res 2019;10(6):336–44.

26. Sharma D, Shah A, Osten M, et al. Efficacy and safety of the GuideLiner Mother-in-Child guide catheter extension in percutaneous coronary intervention. J Interv Cardiol 2017;30(1):46–55.

27. Tsujimura T, Ishihara T, Iida O, et al. Successful percutaneous retrieval of a detached microcatheter tip using the guide-extension catheter trapping technique: A case report. J Cardiol Cases 2019; 20(5):168–71.

28. Desai CK, Petrasko M, Steffen K, et al. Retained coronary balloon requiring emergent open surgical

retrieval: an uncommon complication requiring individualized management strategies. Methodist Debakey Cardiovasc J 2019;15(1):81–5.

29. Utsunomiya M, Kobayashi T, Nakamura S. Case of dislodged stent lost in septal channel during stent delivery in complex chronic total occlusion of right coronary artery. J Invasive Cardiol 2009;21(11): E229–33.

30. Alomar ME, Michael TT, Patel VG, et al. Stent loss and retrieval during percutaneous coronary interventions: a systematic review and meta-analysis. J Invasive Cardiol 2013;25(12):637–41.

31. Brilakis ES, Best PJ, Elesber AA, et al. Incidence, retrieval methods, and outcomes of stent loss during percutaneous coronary intervention: a large single-center experience. Catheter Cardiovasc Interv 2005;66(3):333–40.

32. Malik SA, Brilakis ES, Pompili V, et al. Lost and found: coronary stent retrieval and review of literature. Catheter Cardiovasc Interv 2018;92(1): 50–3.

33. Ritchie JL, Hansen DD, Intlekofer MJ, et al. Rotational approaches to atherectomy and thrombectomy. Z Kardiol 1987;76(Suppl 6):59–65.

34. Kaneda H, Saito S, Hosokawa G, et al. Trapped Rotablator: kokesi phenomenon. Catheter Cardiovasc Interv 2000;49(1):82–4 [discussion: 85].

35. Imamura S, Nishida K, Kawai K, et al. A rare case of Rotablator((R)) driveshaft fracture and successful percutaneous retrieval of a trapped burr using a balloon and GuideLiner((R)). Cardiovasc Interv Ther 2017;32(3):294–8.

36. Tomey MI, Kini AS, Sharma SK. Current status of rotational atherectomy. JACC Cardiovasc Interv 2014;7(4):345–53.

37. Cunnington M, Egred M. GuideLiner, a child-in-a-mother catheter for successful retrieval of an entrapped rotablator burr. Catheter Cardiovasc Interv 2012;79(2):271–3.

38. Kanazawa T, Kadota K, Mitsudo K. Successful rescue of stuck rotablator burr entrapment using a Kiwami straight catheter. Catheter Cardiovasc Interv 2015;86(5):942–5.

39. Sakakura K, Ako J, Momomura S. Successful removal of an entrapped rotablation burr by extracting drive shaft sheath followed by balloon dilatation. Catheter Cardiovasc Interv 2011;78(4): 567–70.

40. Prasan AM, Patel M, Pitney MR, et al. Disassembly of a rotablator: getting out of a trap. Catheter Cardiovasc Interv 2003;59(4):463–5.

41. Brilakis E. Chapter 6 - The retrograde approach. In: Brilakis E, editor. Manual of chronic total occlusion interventions. 2nd Edition. Academic Press; 2018. p. 197–251.

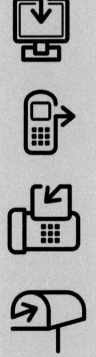
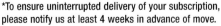